Improving Learning in Uganda Vol. 1

Community-Led School Feeding Practices

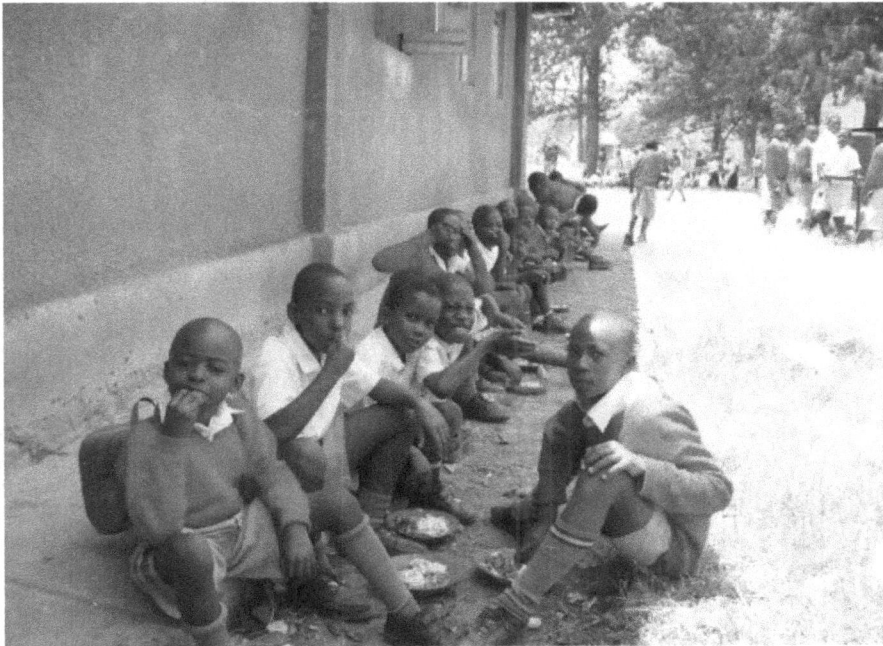

Innocent Mulindwa Najjumba, Charles Lwanga Bunjo,
David Kyaddondo, and Cyprian Misinde

THE WORLD BANK
Washington, D.C.

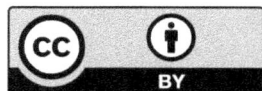

Contents

Boxes

Figures

Foreword

The past one and a half decades have seen many school systems in Africa expand through the introduction of mass education reforms. To achieve those reforms, countries are currently grappling to improve the quality of service delivery by providing key inputs such as qualified teachers, instructional materials, more relevant and child-friendly curriculum, and enhanced infrastructure. However, efficient use of those key inputs can be realized only if learners are able and motivated to learn.

Uganda has been at the forefront of this reform process, but it now finds that—with 92 percent of rural children reporting to school without breakfast and with more than 70 percent spending the school day without lunch—there may be a missing element in realizing the desired outcomes. Children who are hungry or unhealthy or both cannot learn, because hunger and ill health work as disincentives for children to attend and complete school.

Reforms that are grounded on a sound assessment of the country's situation, together with well-elaborated partnership norms for parents and communities, have a high potential for success—but only if the government provides an enabling environment for all key players to effectively participate. Uganda's population is 80 percent rural and is engaged in subsistence farming. Moreover, recent national statistics indicate that only 4 percent of households report food shortages. The hunger of schoolchildren does not then reflect a problem about food security; thus, it should be possible to leverage this potential and to achieve sustainable solutions to the school feeding challenge.

Uganda's political economy celebrates the central role of parents in ensuring child development. The analyses described in this book underscore the potential for Uganda to unleash the power of this legislated partnership with parents by removing some of the barriers that currently prevent parents from realizing their full potential to play a role in feeding their children at school.

Through an analysis of direct observation of sparsely spread school experiences, together with an examination of the cost implications for a national school feeding program, the report highlights various school feeding options that could be made available for parents to adopt through a sustained and school-led dialogue that is enabled by clear policy guidance about the roles and responsibilities of duty bearers at various levels. The results of the analyses of the strengths and weaknesses of each modality emphasize the need to think beyond a single modality and instead to recognize the need for multiple approaches that reflect the socioeconomic and cultural heterogeneity across households and geographical zones in Uganda.

The report also recognizes that school feeding not only addresses education needs, but also has the potential to provide a productive safety net. To achieve this potential, one needs to target programs at the extremely poor and those vulnerable to exclusion. If they are well targeted, the school feeding programs could help children realize their right to education through cost-effective and sustainable modalities. Taking this approach to school feeding would also provide the country with an opportunity to adapt and implement ongoing regional programs—such as the Home-Grown School Feeding approach—which have far-reaching effects in regard to raising household and community incomes that accrue from feeding children at school.

This report makes clear that the national debate about school feeding would benefit from refocusing. For example, the question is not whether parents should or should not pay for school feeding because all approaches involve a cost to parents; even the seemingly free models such as food packing have significant costs. The real question is what is the most effective way for parents to participate in supporting school feeding that, in turn, benefits the education of their children. The report also emphasizes the emerging role for government to support parental efforts with complementary programs such as deworming and other school health initiatives.

One hopes that these analyses about Uganda and the lessons presented from other settings will enable Uganda to move to a more strategic and sustainable approach to school feeding—an approach that would be founded on a strong partnership with parents and communities and would be complemented by the government's health-promoting programs and support to the most vulnerable identified through well-designed and efficiently delivered modalities. This presentation is among the first analyses in Africa to examine how parents and communities have themselves taken up the challenge of feeding their children during the school day. It carries important messages for all the countries throughout Africa and beyond that are seeking to develop sustainable, community-led school feeding programs.

Donald A. P. Bundy
Lead Specialist
Africa Region Technical Health
World Bank

Acknowledgments

This work benefited from financial support from the United Kingdom's Department for International Development (DFID) Trust Fund for the Implementation of the National Development Plan.

The primary author of this report, Innocent Najjumba Mulindwa, Education Specialist, World Bank, extends appreciation to Charles Lwanga Bunjo, David Kyaddondo, and Cyprian Misinde (Consultants), who undertook the field work for the study on community-led school feeding practices, which was commissioned and led by the World Bank; and hence coauthors of this report. The district-specific reports can be accessed from the World Bank. Special appreciation is extended to Clarence Tsimpo Nkengne, economist, World Bank, for technical support in the analysis for the excluded groups.

From the concept note stage to finalization, useful technical comments and encouragement were received from Donald Bundy, lead specialist, and Andy Chi Tembon, coordinator, Africa Region Technical Health Unit, World Bank, who also reviewed the survey tools and initial drafts of this work. The report also benefited from the technical input and guidance of Marcelo Becerra, Carla Bertoncino, Kamel Braham, Sukhdeep Brar, Susan Hirshberg, and Cristina Romero of the World Bank. Strategic and timely guidance from Peter Materu and Moustapha A. Ndiaye was valuable.

Extremely helpful was the valuable support received from the government of Uganda's counterpart team of the Ministry of Education and Sports, most especially from Richard Kabagambe, Aggrey Kibenge, Cathbert Mulyalya, and Daniel Nkaada, who were under the leadership of Permanent Secretary F. X. Lubanga. Support from James Muwonge, Uganda Bureau of Statistics (especially in regard to accessing the 2009/10 Uganda National Panel Survey data), is also highly appreciated. The timely administrative support of Agnes Kaye, together with Emily Wakiuru Mwai of the World Bank, was complemented by the headquarters oversight from Bee Pang. Appreciation is also extended to the DFID Trust Fund management team consisting of Kasper Dalten, former Trust Fund Manager, and Catherine Ssekimpi, current Trust Fund Manager, who were regularly contacted about funding aspects of this work.

About the Authors

Innocent Mulindwa Najjumba is education specialist in the World Bank, currently co-task managing the Bank education portfolio in Uganda. She is a trained demographer and educator, with a working experience spanning education (all sub sectors), local governance, and development assistance, together with emergency programming. She also has vast research experience on Uganda with special focus on HIV and AIDS, chronic poverty, adolescent reproductive health, disability and gender. Current research efforts on education have centered on issues affecting quality education service delivery, particularly school based management, school feeding, teacher effectiveness and learning outcomes. She received her Ph.D in population studies from Makerere University.

Lwanga Bunjo Charles is a lecturer of demographic methods at Makerere University currently pursuing a doctoral degree at the Northwest University-Mafikeng Campus of South Africa. He is a trained statistician with extensive experience in designing social surveys, managing large data sets and undertaking analyses with application of various statistical models. His current research interests are in the area of family demography working on the implications of cohabitation for marriage, marital stability and fertility in Uganda with application of event history analysis methods.

David Kyaddondo is a senior lecturer at Makerere University and an affiliated researcher with the child health and development center. This is a multi-disciplinary institution fostering national capacity building for child survival and development. His research experiences spans health, HIV and AIDS, household dynamics, food security, child nutrition and partnerships for health. Future research interests include health systems and community health management processes. He received a Ph.D. in Anthropology from the University of Copenhagen.

Cyprian Misinde is an assistant lecturer of population studies at Makerere University, currently pursuing a doctoral degree at the Queen's University Belfast. He has trained in population and development with experience in social research. He is currently conducting research on child poverty.

Abbreviations

AIDS	acquired immune deficiency syndrome
CHISOM	Child Support Organisation Mpigi
CSB	corn-soya blend
DEO	District Education Officer
DFID	Department of Internal Development (United Kingdom)
DIS	District Inspector of Schools
EMIS	Education Management Information System
FAO	Food and Agriculture Organisation
FFA	Food for Assets
FRESH	Focusing Resources for Effective School Health
GoU	government of Uganda
HIV	human immunodeficiency virus
MoES	Ministry of Education and Sports
MVP	Millennium Village Project
NDP	National Development Plan
PMT	proxy means testing
PTA	Parents and Teachers Association
QEI	Quality Enhancement Initiative
SMC	School Management Committee
SOCADIDO	social development nongovernmental organization of the Catholic Church
SWOT	strengths, weaknesses, opportunities, threats
THR	take-home rations
UNESCO	United Nations Educational, Scientific, and Cultural Organization
UNHS	Uganda National Household Survey
UNICEF	United Nations Children's Fund

UPE	Universal Primary Education
UPPET	Uganda Post-Primary Education and Training
WFP	World Food Programme
WHO	World Health Organization

Monetary

| U Sh | Uganda shilling |
| US$ | U.S. dollar |

Executive Summary

At the launch of the Universal Primary Education (UPE) program in 1997 in Uganda, roles and responsibilities of key players in providing education were identified and eventually amplified in the Education (Pre-Primary, Primary, and Post-Primary) Act of 2008. Under this law, the government provides inputs through capitation grant allocations to schools, instructional materials, and infrastructural support, while providing food is one of the responsibilities left to parents and school communities. Home-packed meals have been the government's recommended and promoted school feeding modality, most importantly for rural schools that register 80 percent of the estimated 7.9 million learners in primary schools, but that recommendation has had minimal success.

According to the 2009/10 Uganda National Household Survey (UNHS), 92 percent of rural children who attend primary school do not have breakfast at home, and about 7 in every 10 day scholars in public schools spend the day without lunch, which undoubtedly has a negative impact on their readiness and ability to learn. A learner who is "motivated and ready to learn" is one of the core elements of an effective teaching-learning process. Addressing this challenge is, therefore, central to the quality education enhancement agenda being pursued in Uganda today. The ongoing strategy of the World Food Programme (WFP) in assisting the government of Uganda (GoU) is targeted at only the Karamoja region, which is highly food insecure and educationally disadvantaged.

The policy to devolve school feeding to parents under the UPE program is, on the whole, justifiable. Uganda's population is 81 percent rural and is engaged in subsistence agriculture; three out of every four households have land, and only 4 percent of households are threatened by food shortages and famine (UBOS 2010). Uganda also registers the lowest proportion of the population (5–20 percent) below the minimum level of dietary energy consumption (food deprived) in the eastern and central Africa regions (FAO 2008), while the poverty head count has substantially reduced from 56 percent in 1992 to 24 percent in 2009/10. Those statistics, however, substantially negate the oft-cited rationale for parental failure to provide food to children.

The more likely contributor could be the negative politicization of the universal education reforms in Uganda at all levels, which emphasizes the free nature of the programs with lesser emphasis on the roles of parents, including consistent reinforcement that schools should not be asking for any contribution. In regard to school feeding, for example, rural parents and school administration are limited to only one modality: food packing without consideration for other options that could also be convenient or affordable.

A few schools were reported to be trying to mobilize parents to fulfill this obligation but with a dearth of either documented experiences to inform sector policy discourse or lessons learned from other schools. That lack of information was the main rationale for this analytical work. This report, therefore, attempts to explore ongoing community-led initiatives for school feeding and how those initiatives are implemented at the school level, including operational challenges, which are based on field experiences from selected schools across the country and which inform replication elsewhere. Also presented are issues that the government needs to consider for a sustainable way forward on school feeding in Uganda.

Study Methodology and Scope

The study was undertaken in 11 districts of Uganda. Nine districts were randomly selected on the basis of the regional cluster sampling frame of the Uganda Bureau of Statistics: Amolator, Busia, Bukedea, Kabale, Kayunga, Kibaale, Maracha Mpigi, and Nakapiripirit. Two more districts were purposively selected: Kampala district, because of its unique and metropolitan nature, and Isingiro district, for the ongoing Millennium Village Project (MVP), which encompasses a school feeding scheme.

This study adopted a case study survey design to enable comprehensive understanding of implementation modalities of ongoing school feeding practices. It has a broader objective of identifying good practices that would inform the next steps in school feeding in Uganda. The respective school feeding options thus served as case studies. Data collection methodologies that were used included desk reviews, focus group discussions, key informant interviews, narratives, and observational techniques. School selection was guided by information from District Education Officers (DEOs) and District Inspectors of Schools (DISs). More than 10 schools per district were visited, but only 3 per district were selected for detailed study on the basis of (a) the willingness of the school administration to participate in the survey and (b) the scale and viability of respective school feeding operations. Schools were visited at least twice to validate the information collected through interviews with observations.

Results

The following school feeding options were observed in schools but had very limited coverage: (a) home-packed food, (b) hot meals prepared by schools, and (c) food vending or school canteens. The summary that follows in table O.1 provides operational modalities of the respective modalities, including strengths, weaknesses, and success factors.

Table O.1 Summary of Existing Community-Led Practices

Strengths/opportunities	Weaknesses	Success factors based on good practices

Option I: Home-Packed Meals—Locally known as *entanda*, this option involves the carrying of packed food from home by learners for consumption at school during the midmorning, at lunch breaks, or both. It is also the most promoted option by the government and the only approach recommended for rural schools—as reported by district and school personnel.

Strengths/opportunities	Weaknesses	Success factors based on good practices
• Is relatively less exclusive. • Is easier to promote because it is an older practice. • Is easy to manage by school because it is household led. • Ensures the full engagement of parents in the well-being of children. • Promotes household cautiousness to food security.	• It depends on availability of food at the household level. • It is sensitive to the type of staple food and sociocultural factors. • The food standard setting is difficult as a result of household heterogeneity. • It is more acceptable to lower primary children and to girls than to upper-primary children and boys. • It is difficult to ensure parental compliance.	• Sustained mobilization in the community. • Food type: not all staples are eligible for packing. • School level norms that enhance parental adherence. • Parental commitment. • Food availability at the household level, which is: either leftover or easily prepared food or snacks.

Option II: Hot Meals at School—Hot food is enabled through **voluntary arrangements** with parents and the community to make either in-kind food contributions or cash contributions to facilitate food availability and preparation. Outputs from school gardens are in some instances also used to feed children.

1. **Use of in-kind food contributions by parents** is practiced mostly in rural areas. Average quantity contributed per child is 13 kilograms and 8 kilograms of maize and beans, respectively, for solid meals and 5 kilograms of maize for semisolid meals (porridge). Cash contribution is also required to enable food processing (milling) and preparation.

2. **Use of cash contributions by parents** is overtly practiced in urban schools and covertly practiced in the rural schools. Average contribution per child per term in rural schools was U Sh 6,500/= for semisolid meals (19,500 per year) and 20,000/= (60,000 per year) for solid meals, with significant variations across districts.

3. **Use of school gardens** is practiced in rural schools where land size and ownership norms allow. Gardening is done by pupils either during agriculture lessons or any other time agreed to by the school administration.

Strengths/opportunities	Weaknesses	Success factors based on good practices

• A hot meal is highly desirable by parents and school management teams because
  - It enhances parental and community support to education as a result of high and regular stakeholder engagement.
  - It enables emergence of school-level institutional structures for promoting student welfare.
  - It ensures uniformity of food quality, quantity, and type, and it reduces differentiation among learners.
  - It increases school attendance.
• A hot meal boosts community and household incomes through local food purchases and processing by the school.
• A hot meal provides opportunities for line sectors to participate in school activities (for example, tree-planting campaigns by the environment sector, promotion of high-yield seeds for school gardens by the agriculture sector, high-value food preparation modalities by the health sector, etc.
• School gardens enhance learner knowledge and skills in farming; they also provide avenues for introducing new crop varieties to the community.
	• It is exclusionary in nature because eligibility is determined by the ability of parents to contribute.
	• It imposes indirect costs on the school management, compounded by ever-rising food prices.
	• School-level requirements for fuel (firewood, charcoal) impose environmental challenges for the school and community.
	• A lack of school kitchens, water, and serving facilities will constrain operations.
		• Functional and effective institutional framework for sustained mobilization and participation of the community.
		• Hygienic school environments such as water, food storage, and cooking facilities, including serving areas.
		• Cooking utensils and labor to support food preparation.
		• Proper records management for building trust, transparency and accountability.
		• Nonparticipation (direct) in food preparation by teachers and learners.

(table continues on next page)

Table O.1 Summary of Existing Community-Led Practices (continued)

Strengths/opportunities	Weaknesses	Success factors based on good practices
Option II: Food Vending and School Canteen—This option involves selling and buying of food items by community members and learners, respectively, from spaces provided by the school administration. Participation of learners depends on their ability to pay for what is being sold. Average minimum cost for one item is 500/=.		
• Has minimal responsibility for school management. • Is less prone to political interference. • Boosts community incomes because suppliers are within the community. • Complements other school-feeding options.	• Poor food-handling practices compromise food quality. • There is limited control over sources and quality of vended food by school. • This option is expensive for the low-income households; an estimated minimum per child per year is U Sh 120,000/=. • There is a potential for parental exploitation if the schools do not regulate maximum charges for items sold. • This option interferes with schooling if teachers and pupils are also involved in food vending.	• Complements other school feeding options. • Has limiting direct involvement of teachers and pupils. • Covers clearly gazetted food vending sites at school with erected food vending stands to maintain basic hygiene standards.

Source: World Bank data.

Issues for the Government to Consider

The low coverage of initiatives, especially in rural schools, deserves attention. Rural schools are limited to home-packed food because the schools have no space for other options, however desirable, which further widens the urban-rural schooling gap. Therefore, the key question that remains is this: how do schools meaningfully engage parents to provide food to children in accordance with what is considered desirable and convenient to them?

Schools need a menu of school feeding options to enable flexibility and responsiveness to social, cultural, and other contextual factors involving learners. Opening space for additional options should be considered with harmonization and standardization of implementation modalities done at the district level for optimal benefits and sustainable evolution of effective and efficient community-led and parent-led programs.

The government should refocus the debate on school feeding. The focus of the debate on school feeding has been more on (a) the mandatory nature of requiring parents to pack food for their children, and (b) the illegal nature of especially parents' cash contributions to schools under the universal education programs. It is evident that all school feeding options have a cost attached to them. The government should thus give full autonomy to School Management

Committees (SMCs) and the school administration to generate a consensus among parents. The government should provide support to SMCs and should lead this dialogue by issuing guidelines that clarify possible options that the schools could consider, including the roles of key players and institutional setup.

Financial implications of a national school feeding program deserve attention for informed decision making at all levels. Costs of school feeding vary by country, but a regional study (The Gambia, Kenya, Lesotho, and Malawi) put costs at an average of US$40 per child per year, while the World Food Programme (WFP) average annual estimate is US$50 per child. Those costs translate into an average annual requirement of at least US$218 million for a national school feeding program for Uganda. The draft Cabinet Memo on School Feeding by the Ministry of Education and Sports (MoES) estimated U Sh 100 per child, which translates to U Sh 24,000 (US$9.60) per child per year and hence an average of US$52.4 million per year. Of importance to note is that this estimate is about 75 percent lower than the regional average and 25 percent lower than the head teachers' and DEOs' estimated average of U Sh 30,000 (US$11) per child per year, yet it is 3.5 times higher than the annual primary education capitation per child in Uganda! Any financing decisions by the government, therefore, must be realistic, and the sustainability commitment has to be guaranteed over time. Dangers of unrealistic contributions include raising expectations, creating a relentless demand for more from parents, and suppressing community and school innovations.

The government's responding to household shocks and targeting the excluded is necessary as an incentive for those who have been excluded to attend and complete school. School feeding not only is valuable for educational gains but also is a social protection strategy. The identified options are all household driven, thus are prone to excluding learners from households affected by various socioeconomic and environmental shocks. Government needs to consider other targeting modalities for school feeding elsewhere, in addition to the ongoing WFP/GoU program by focusing on the food insecure and educationally disadvantaged Karamoja region. This strategy, however, calls for the design of various targeting modalities including geographical (regional and district) and proxy means testing (PMT), according to which the excluded could be effectively identified and reached.

Community-led school feeding also needs planning for sustainability. The decision to devolve this function to parents and communities was visionary and places Uganda high on the sustainability continuum. This devolution is, however, affected by a lack of clarity and openness, thereby leading to a weak partnership with parents and resulting in nonexecution of their roles. All options need planning for sustainability either by parents or by the school administration. Clear and realistic school-level feeding plans are thus necessary but can exist only if school management is granted full autonomy and clear guidance on the various options available.

School-level operational arrangements deserve attention too. The multiplicity of players in the community-led school feeding options is evident, which is commendable and positive for sustainability purposes. Roles vary by player and in some instances by respective school feeding option. School-level institutional structures that engage all players need to be put in place to ensure effective coordination and implementation.

Accountability and procurement monitoring systems are crucial for the smooth running of community-led school feeding programs. Opening up school feeding programs to other options has accountability challenges that deserve attention to avoid abuse and eventual mistrust among players. Transparent, flexible—but not complex—processes should be instituted that include all players for trust and partnership building. School procurements from the community have the potential to develop local food production and processing capacities and to provide schools with a potential for price negotiations and maximum value for resources. Using experience from parents' infrastructure contributions, schools may be mandated with guidance from MoES to evolve simple, transparent, and satisfactory procurement and accountability systems for food-related aspects of education.

School-level infrastructure is insufficient. Lack of physical facilities to support food storage, food preparation, and related activities was noted in all schools visited, which compromises food quality and hygiene standards. The MoES needs to develop low-cost infrastructure designs for schools to adopt. It will also guide their resource mobilization drives.

Improvements in food value and hygiene standards are required. Unbalanced meals characterized by solid bulky starch with low protein and fat were observed, with the limited coverage of operations notwithstanding. Vegetables and fruits were not seen even in the vending places. Low food hygiene standards were also observed across the board: there were no storage areas, cooking and eating places were inadequate and unclean, vending areas were dirty, and there was no water or soap for hand washing. Training in food value and hygiene is, therefore, important for all players. In Ghana, the training provided by the health sector for all cooks helped improve this area, including identification and treatment of those with communicable diseases.

Complementary approaches are necessary for healthy learners. Deworming, nutritional supplementation (vitamin A, iron, and zinc), and food fortification are important in the control and prevention of micronutrient deficiencies among learners. These approaches are also recommended by the United Nations Educational, Scientific, and Cultural Organization (UNESCO) and the World Health Organization (WHO). In Kenya, deworming alone reduced absenteeism by 25 percent; Tanzania and Cambodia use food fortification powder at the school cooking sites with the support of the government and the ministry of health. Implementation of these interventions through schools has been found to be very cost-effective and safe. Such programs could be considered in Uganda as one of the government's contributions in partnership with agencies such as the United Nations Children's Fund (UNICEF) and WHO.

Environmental concerns prevail. Expanding school feeding operations poses significant environmental concerns, especially regarding deforestation. Promotion of fuel-saving cooking technologies and tree planting in schools is important. Links with line sectors are necessary, including promotion of fuel-saving designs of stoves and cooking areas.

Monitoring and evaluating community-led school feeding practices are equally important. To amplify visibility of such operations, they need to be mainstreamed in the Education Management Information System (EMIS). Clear and measurable indicators need to be developed, which is also central to the sustainability aspect.

Political will is central to the promotion and scaling-up of community-led school feeding initiatives in Uganda. The current rating for Uganda's political will to promote community-based school feeding schemes would be considered low. Messages and actions from political leadership at all levels should thus be in support of these schemes. Technocrats also need to guarantee that all regulatory instruments and other elements are in place to guide and ensure quality implementation of these initiatives.

Possible Strategic Actions

Action 1. *Removing all barriers to parental participation to enable schools have a menu of school feeding options that are sensitive to regional and household heterogeneity, as well as a sustainable partnership.* Feeding all children by government through a well-coordinated and sustainably resourced national school feeding program is not feasible. For example, reasonable funding levels for a national school feeding program would call for an increase in the education sector budget of at least 10.7 percent per annum; while ideal school feeding standards based on regional norms require at least US$218.5 million per annum. The current resource constraints interfaced with other unfunded education priorities may not allow this.

Action 2. *Targeting those children who are excluded as a result of extreme poverty, food insecurity, and household shocks to foster the safety net role of school feeding.* All the observed community-led school feeding options depend on the status of households and hence have an inherent element of exclusion because households are prone to many socioeconomic shocks. In this regard, various modalities of targeting the excluded could be adopted.

Action 3. *Designing and implementing a school health program package aimed at provision of complementary school based health programs such as deworming, and food fortification; reinforced by community and parental training on nutritional values of various foods.* Integration of complementary interventions such as deworming and micronutrient supplementation has potential to augment educational benefits, because good health and nutrition are prerequisites for effective learning.

Recommendations for Next Steps

Adoption of the above mentioned actions calls for the following immediate steps by the Education Sector.

1. Initiate dialogue with government to obtain political buy in on the above mentioned actions.
2. Finalize the draft school feeding guidelines with more clarity on the various school feeding options available to schools for consideration by parents.
3. Distribute and disseminate the guidelines for wider reach and immediate adoption.
4. Form an interministerial committee on school feeding to enable the design and implementation of complementary initiatives as well as school feeding programs for the children likely to be excluded. Expediting passage of the draft School Health Policy would greatly enhance this process.

CHAPTER 1

Introduction

Uganda has registered tremendous success in the expansion of the school system arising from the ongoing Universal Primary Education (UPE) reform that was launched in 1997. Primary enrollment is estimated at 8.7 million children, resulting in a net enrollment ratio of 83.2 percent (UBOS 2010). Completion and achievement rates are, however, still low. More than half the primary pupils in grades 3 and 6 perform below the desired minimum average (50 percent) for numeracy and literacy, while the primary completion rate stands at about 50 percent. By 2007, survival to primary 7 (P7; percentage of a pupil cohort that reaches the end of the primary cycle) was estimated at only 28 percent. The government is thus faced with the dual challenge of maintaining high enrollment levels and ensuring quality service delivery for the realization of national development goals and Millennium Development Goals on education. Government and development partners' efforts are currently focused on improving the provision of key inputs for quality teaching and learning processes—especially qualified teachers, instructional materials, and curriculum reforms—reinforced by school infrastructure developments to support the expansion. However, school-level aspects that continue to feature in the education sector dialogue as constraints to quality learning need to be looked at, the most important being schoolchildren going hungry because of lack of organized school feeding schemes, low capacity of School Management Committees (SMCs), and low quality of teaching-learning processes.

With support from the United Kingdom Department for International Development, the World Bank initiated exploratory analytical work under the broader theme of "improving learning in Uganda," with a specific focus on some of the frequently cited barriers to the realization of quality education service delivery, including school feeding. This analytical work focuses on exploring operational modalities and challenges faced by school administrations in promoting school feeding in Uganda. The report concludes with key issues for government consideration in promoting and scaling up community-led school feeding schemes for improved learning in Uganda.

Background and Rationale

At the launch of the UPE in 1997, roles and responsibilities of key players in providing education were identified and eventually amplified in the Education (Pre-Primary, Primary, and Post-Primary) Act of 2008. Under this law, the government provides inputs through capitation grant allocations to schools, instructional materials, and infrastructural support. Community and family contributions toward the education of children are clearly articulated in article 13c of the act, including provision of food. In essence, the food provision was left in the hands of parents, and school communities are free to establish feeding modalities that are independent of the formal school system.

Because financial contributions from parents to schools are prohibited under the UPE, promotion of home-packed meals has been the government-recommended modality, but it has met with minimal success. This lack of success has been attributed to a number of factors, ranging from lack of food and packing materials at the household level to low appreciation of the links between morning and midday meals and learning outcomes by various responsible parties. Nevertheless, designing effective school-based programs requires an evidence base that provides management teams with information about various feeding options that are based on context, potential benefits, and estimated costs (Bundy et al. 2009), which this analysis attempts to address.

Learner absenteeism in Uganda is high. One of every three children in primary school does not attend school every day (see figure 1.1). Low attendance affects learning and hinders effective use of educational inputs, with a resultant negative

Figure 1.1 Learner Absenteeism by Grade, UNPS 2009/10

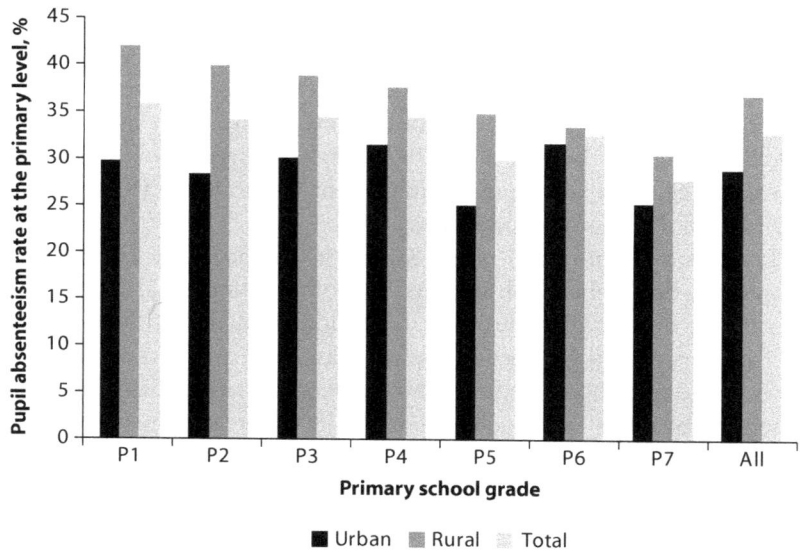

Source: Data from the Uganda Bureau of Statistics.

impact on learning outcomes. For example, going by the 33 percent pupil absenteeism rate at the primary level, we can estimate that Uganda loses at least U Sh 18.2 billion (US$7 million) annually arising from just the direct per capita allocations to schools, which compounds inefficiency. Attendance is an important element of school success, and the literature points to a positive correlation between students' attendance and learning outcomes (Coates 2003; Gottfried 2009). Other research has supported the notion that student attendance records can serve as direct signals to school quality (Coutts 1998). Low attendance rates have thus been cited as detrimental to learning and academic achievement. Students who do not attend school as frequently receive fewer hours of classroom instruction and consequently perform more poorly. Finn (1989) found that consistently low levels of attendance in early grades were associated with higher future academic risks, including nonpromotion and dropout. Irregular attendance of learners was also cited by head teachers as one of the most serious problems faced by schools (25 percent; see figure 1.2). Uganda's education quality enhancement efforts, therefore, need to pay closer attention to some of the contributing factors to low school attendance from the learners' side, in addition to the ongoing improvements in providing key inputs to learning for a holistic approach.

The results of the 2009/10 Uganda National Panel Survey indicate that 73 percent of day scholars attending public primary schools were spending the school day without lunch, and a substantial number were reporting to school without breakfast, which compromises their motivation and readiness to learn right from the start of the school day and over time decreases gains from education investments. The proportion without breakfast was highest in

Figure 1.2 Most Serious Problems Faced by Schools as Identified by Headteachers, UNPS 2009/10

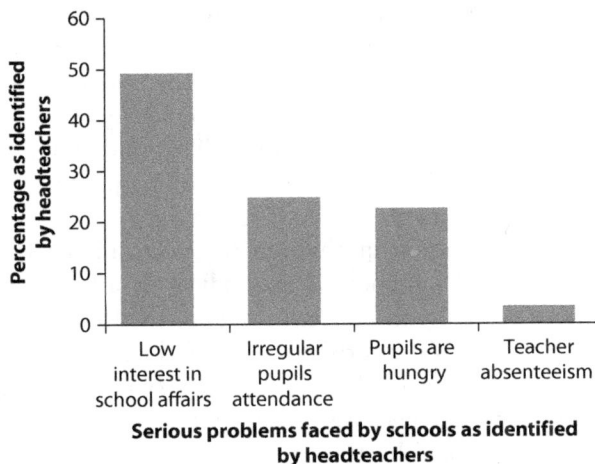

Source: Data from the Uganda Bureau of Statistics.

Figure 1.3 Children 6–12, Who Are in Primary School and Had No Breakfast, UNHS 2009/10

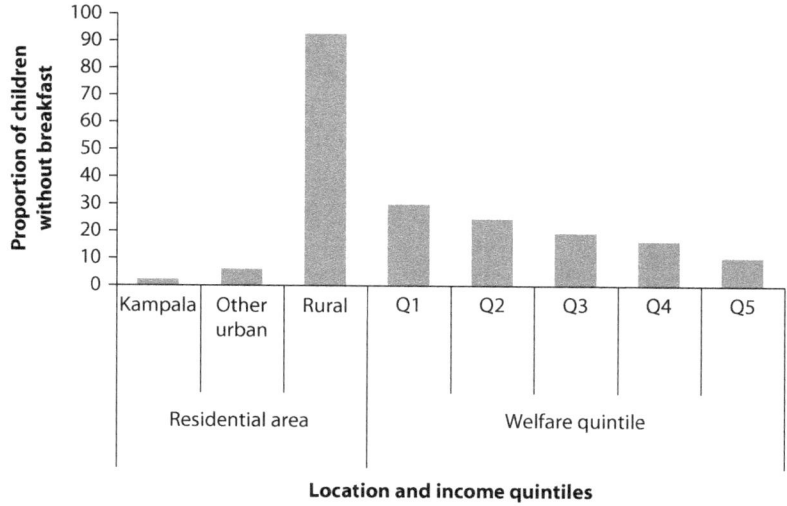

Source: Data from the Uganda Bureau of Statistics.

the rural areas at 92 percent (whereas urban areas had only 5.8 percent going without breakfast), and it declines as one moves from the lowest to highest income quintiles (figure 1.3). A school-based survey conducted in the 12 districts of Uganda implementing the Quality Enhancement Initiative (QEI) also revealed that a majority of learners report to school without breakfast (figure 1.4). The proportion that reported having had breakfast before going to school was highest in Kyenjojo and Mubende districts (44 percent), followed by Lyantonde district (42 percent) and Amuru district (35 percent). The Karamoja districts reported the lowest rates of children who go to school having had breakfast at home: Kaabong (6 percent) and Nakapiripirit (7 percent). Although the low incidence reported in the Karamoja region's districts can be attributed to the low food availability in the region, other districts are expected to have regular food at the household level and should have performed far better than the reported levels. This finding compromises one of the core elements of an effective teaching-learning process: "a learner who is motivated and ready to learn."

Temporary hunger, common in children who are not fed before going to school or in the course of a school day, can adversely affect learning. Hungry children have more difficulty in concentrating and performing complex tasks, even if they are, in fact, well nourished. The World Food Programme (WFP 2006) affirms that when hungry children enroll, they are more likely to either drop out or perform poorly because of intermittent school attendance. Even when they make it to school, short-term hunger arising from missing breakfast or walking long distances to school on empty stomachs affects their attention

Figure 1.4 Percentage of Pupils Who Get Breakfast at Home; QEI Baseline, Uganda 2009

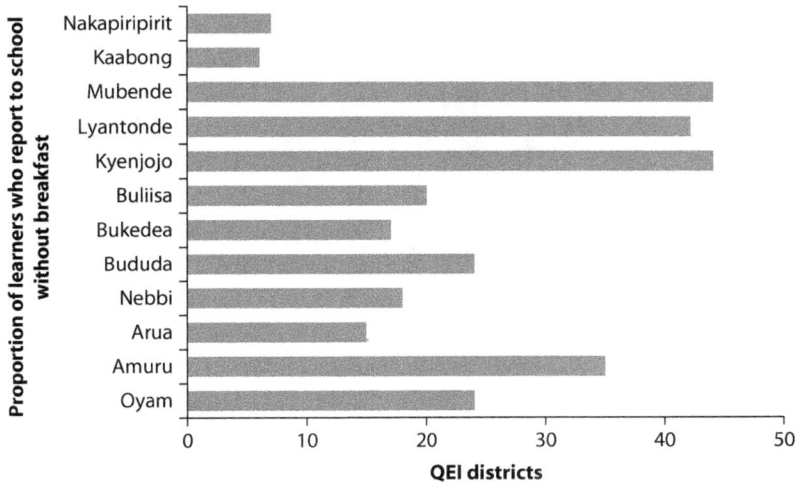

Source: Data from Quality Enhancement Initiative Baseline Survey, Uganda.

span and eventually their overall school performance. In a study about school feeding in Peru and the United States, Pollitt, Cueto, and Jacoby (1998) found that when 9–11-year-old children had not eaten in the morning, they were slower in memory recall and made more errors on tests. Other studies indicate that children who skip breakfast are less able to solve simple visual tasks. On the whole, the preceding findings for Uganda indicate that more than half the children report to school without having had breakfast, which profoundly compromises learning. This finding also points to the extensive efforts that have to be undertaken in a bid to sensitize parents and guardians—as well as the wider community—about the importance of food to learning.

Figures 1.5 and 1.6 further show that teachers consider lack of food one of the causes of learner absenteeism. Of note, teachers perceive the effect of food on learner absenteeism to predominate among lower-primary (47 percent for girls and 44 percent for boys) rather than upper-primary (27 percent for girls and 26 percent for boys) learners. Inspection reports from primary schools indicate that lack of food at school partly contributes to irregular learner attendance. Other issues cited that were linked to lack of food at school include early closures of schools and hence less contact time between learners and teachers with implications on curriculum coverage and learner performance. School-community tensions as hungry children rummage through gardens in search of food either in the morning or at lunch breaks or even after school on their way home also feature in the district inspection reports.

In Uganda, the WFP has undertaken directly providing food to schools over time, targeting populations within geographical areas that are identified to be most prone to food insecurity. This approach has been done through its School

Figure 1.5 Teachers Who Think That Lack of Food Causes Absenteeism at Lower Primary: QEI Baseline, Uganda 2009

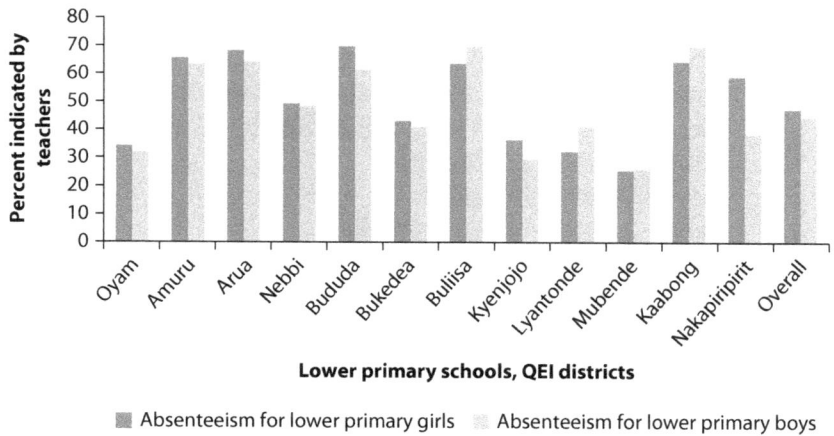

Lower primary schools, QEI districts

■ Absenteeism for lower primary girls   Absenteeism for lower primary boys

Source: Data from Quality Enhancement Initiative Baseline Survey, Uganda.

Figure 1.6 Teachers Who Think That Lack of Meals Causes Absenteeism at Upper Primary: QEI Baseline, Uganda 2009

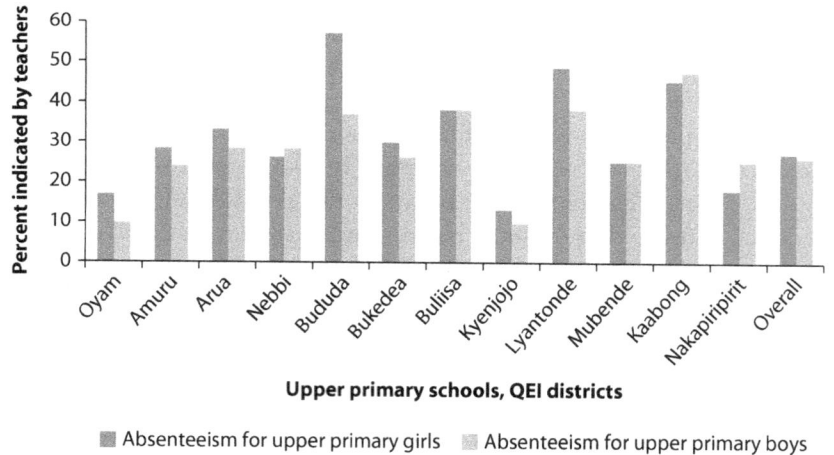

Upper primary schools, QEI districts

■ Absenteeism for upper primary girls   ▓ Absenteeism for upper primary boys

Source: Data from Quality Enhancement Initiative Baseline Survey, Uganda.

Feeding Programs and later Food for Education programs, which were implemented in the conflict areas of northern Uganda and in the Karamoja region, which also had a take-home rations (THR) program for girls.[1]

The Food for Assets (FFA) program, which ran from 2005 to 2007, helped schools in the northern region access key inputs (seeds and farm equipment) and mobilize parents and the wider community to use school land for their school feeding programs according to food harvests. This program was also useful for the revival of school gardens. With the transition from conflict to postconflict and recovery phase in the northern region, WFP food provision was stopped in 2007. Since 2008, the WFP has continued with the Institutional School Meals program only for the Karamoja region because of the region's high food insecurity and poverty. To enable schools to effectively transit from WFP operations to household-supported school feeding for children, the Packed Lunch Campaign was supported in one of the districts (Amuru) with an aim of encouraging parents to send children to school with a packed meal. The initiative was driven by an awareness campaign facilitated by radio programs and community champions and included provision of lunch boxes. Plans to extend this campaign to other districts are constrained by finances.

The expanded school feeding program for Uganda also brought on board the Home-Grown School Feeding program, which was launched in 2005 in partnership with the New Partnership for Africa's Development. The scheme links school feeding directly with agricultural development and promotes buying food and other items for the school feeding program from local farmers. The scheme reduces malnutrition while providing local farmers with the opportunity to sell their produce to participating schools and is one of the good practices that deserve promotion as the government considers developing sustainable school feeding mechanisms. However, this scheme was limited to the WFP program areas.

Ongoing isolated and undocumented school-based interventions deserve an in-depth study to inform the government of possible action areas on this agenda. For example, adding to the WFP school feeding operations highlighted earlier, anecdotal evidence suggests that some effective SMCs and Parents and Teachers Associations (PTAs) have been able to work out modalities that are responsive to context-specific norms, drawing from community strengths and multisectoral program opportunities that exist. In some schools of eastern Uganda, for example, parents contribute corn in kind plus a small fee toward grinding the corn and purchasing auxiliary items used in school kitchens and as wages for cooks, as agreed by respective SMCs and PTAs.

In other areas, school managers have tapped into existing programs such as National Agricultural Advisory Services to revamp school gardens where land size allows, proceeds of which are consumed by learners; while in other settings, innovations such as school canteens were reported to be up and running. However, little is known about school coping mechanisms in their entirety or sustainability, potential risks, and benefits of various coping strategies to the wider community for informed sector dialogue and cohesive policy implementation. Worse still, learners who are spending their school time with empty stomachs are still common in schools, contributing to irregular attendance, ineffective in-school transactions, and low learning outcomes, all of which negate the gains that would have been realized from the education investments made by various stakeholders, including government, development partners, parents, and the wider community.

As articulated by the WFP (2006), addressing both hunger and inadequate learning can lead to improvements in human capital development and greater economic growth, both of which are central to Uganda's National Development Plan (NDP), which makes school feeding of relevance in Uganda today. The need to work out efficient and sustainable modalities of providing food to learners while at school, therefore, continues to dominate the education sector discourse. The fact that a high proportion of learners report to school without breakfast and go without lunch deserves attention.

School Feeding and Learning—Scientific Evidence

Although undernutrition during pregnancy and infancy causes most harm to the long-term learning capacity of individuals through its irreversible damage to the brain structure and size caused by low birth weight, growth faltering, and micronutrient deficiencies, its impact on school-going children also deserves attention. Hunger affects school-going children's ability to make use of opportunities to learn, which likely reduces the gains realized from education investments. School feeding programs, therefore, help get children into school and keep them there by enhancing enrollment and reducing absenteeism; once children are in school, the programs can contribute to children's learning by avoiding their hunger and enhancing their cognitive abilities—especially if complemented by deworming and micronutrients (Ahmed 2004; Bundy et al. 2009). Short-term hunger keeps children out of school and limits their ability to concentrate when there. The short-term effects of providing children with a meal during the school day, therefore, include alleviating hunger and helping them concentrate and learn better, thereby improving school performance.

A meta-analysis undertaken by the WFP on 32 Sub-Saharan Africa countries indicated that school feeding is associated with increased enrollment, especially for girls (Gelli, Meir, and Espejo 2007). In areas with high human immunodeficiency virus (HIV) prevalence, emerging evidence shows that school feeding has the potential of enhancing enrollment, attendance, and progression of orphans and other vulnerable children (Edstrom et al. 2008). A randomized controlled trial on school feeding in Jamaica found that scores in arithmetic improved by 0.11 standard deviation, and the improvement was attributed to the increased frequency and effectiveness with which learners attended school (Jukes, Drake, and Bundy 2008). In rural India, according to school panel survey data, the transition from monthly distribution of free food grains to daily provision of cooked meals to schoolchildren improved monthly attendance of grade 1 learners by 12 percent (Afridi 2010).

Randomized impact evaluation studies conducted in northern Uganda between 2005 and 2007 about the effects of WFP's alternative primary school Food for Education programs revealed that school feeding had a positive effect on learners' cognitive development as reflected in their ability to manipulate concepts (Adelman, Gilligan, and Lehrer 2008). Further research undertaken in the same region indicated that School Feeding Programs and THR provided by the WFP had significant effects on learner attendance, especially for grades 1–2 among boys and 6–7 for the girls (Alderman, Gilligan, and Lehrer 2008). The same study indicated that the school meals program significantly affected afternoon school attendance. In the specification with controls for school quality, the estimated effect of the School Feeding Program was 9.3 percentage points increase in the probability that a child attends school after lunchtime. WFP school-specific reports also indicate that the FFA program, through which parents participated in school gardening to grow food for their children in school, substantially contributed to learning improvements in some schools. For example, Kalaki Primary School in Kaberamaido district reduced the dropout rate by 62 percent and increased enrollment by 40 percent between 2005 and 2007.

Methodology

This analytical work draws from a sample survey on community-led school feeding in Uganda that was commissioned by the World Bank between February and April 2011. A case study design was used, where the different types of feeding practices served as cases for purposes of generating a comprehensive understanding of the respective community-led school feeding options being adopted. Distinctive attributes of each particular feeding approach (case) were examined while paying attention to matters of history, context, physical setting, various actors, range and nature of food, and beneficiaries.

Sampling procedures. This study recognized the country's regional variations in respect to economic situations; agriculture and food crops; cultural practices, including those related to food; and history, all of which might have a bearing on community feeding initiatives. The Uganda Bureau of Statistics regional grouping that clusters the country into 9 regions was used. These groups are Central 1 and 2, Eastern, East-Central, North, North-East, North-West (West Nile), South West, and Western. Kampala was also included as a specific study region because of its special status in terms of population, urban nature, and economic situation. From each of the regions, one district was randomly selected using the rotary method. The process generated the following 10 districts: Amolator, Bukedea, Busia, Kabale, Kampala, Kayunga, Kibaale, Maracha, Mpigi, and Nakapiripirit. In addition to the randomly selected districts, Isingiro district was purposively selected in a bid to capture operations of the ongoing community-based school feeding arrangement implemented under the Millennium Village Project, thereby bringing the total sample of districts to 11.

At the district level, a list of schools with various school feeding practices was obtained from the respective District Education Officers (DEOs) with support from the District Inspector of Schools (DIS). The DEOs did not have comprehensive information about schools by feeding options for children in all the districts visited. Lists of about 25–35 primary schools were provided in each of the districts, from which 10 schools (one-third urban) were visited by the research team with guidance and participation of the DIS. The initial visits to the schools enabled assessment of existing practices in the schools and a decision on whether respective schools qualified for case studies. Of the 10 visited schools, 3 schools per district were finally selected to participate in the survey on the basis of the willingness of the school administration, the viability of the ongoing school feeding practices as indicated by the number of participating pupils, and the type of school feeding option. The respective school feeding options served as cases that were used in this investigation.

Data collection methods. Different qualitative data collection methods were used to obtain and triangulate views from different actors. These methods included the following:

- Desk reviews with specific focus on policy documents for education and other line sectors
- Key informant interviews targeting key stakeholders at the district and school levels (head teachers, teachers, SMC executive members, and student leaders; 73 in total)
- Focus group discussions (17 in total) with pupils participating in a specific school feeding option
- Observational techniques that enabled comprehensive understanding of the processes and other elements such as the food menu, facilities available, dynamics in food provision, school settings under which food is prepared and served to learners, and efficiency issues related to food preparation
- School feeding narratives and case stories from school administrators, parents, and selected children to give detailed description of events, accounts, recounts, experiences, and perspectives of various actors participating in different school feeding activities.

Qualitative data analysis techniques were used to identify emerging themes of relevance to the study. These themes were validated by either existing quantitative data or narrative statements to justify raising the issue. Summaries of the case studies have also been used whenever appropriate with the strengths, weaknesses, opportunities, threats (SWOT) analysis for the respective school feeding options.

The survey was guided by the following questions:

- How do existing policies address the issue of school feeding in Uganda?
- Who is involved and responsible for planning, overseeing, and preparing meals in the different feeding arrangements that prevail in schools?
- What are the forms of community participation and contributions to the different school feeding options?
- How do the regional and local context variations influence the feeding options adopted in different schools?

- What is the type, quality, quantity, and nutritional content of food provided to learners?
- What school feeding practices exist, and are they sustainable?
- Does a particular feeding option have mechanisms for inclusion of vulnerable children (very poor)?
- What were the strengths and weaknesses of various school feeding programs and contexts?
- What feeding options could be replicated or have potential for replication?

Report Structure

This report is divided into four main chapters. Chapter 1 is this introduction. Chapter 2 provides the policy framework for school feeding in Uganda while chapter 3 presents the observed community-led school feeding practices in Uganda. Chapter 4 provides insights on issues for consideration by the government and especially the Ministry of Education and Sports (MoES) to generate a clear way forward for school feeding in Uganda. The report ends with an appendix and a reference list.

Significantly, this analysis did not attempt to assess the effect of community-led school feeding practices in Uganda, nor is it an in-depth study of ongoing development partner-supported initiatives. However, attempts to draw from their experiences and data sources have been made as appropriate.

Note

1. See WFP reports on Uganda.

CHAPTER 2

The National Policy Framework on School Feeding

Uganda has no explicit school feeding policy. However, collaborative discussions between the ministries of health and education yielded the draft National Guidelines on School Feeding of July 2010, drawing from the draft National School Health Policy. The objectives of the guidelines are to (a) guide the planning, selection, handling, preparation, and service of nutritious school meals using locally available foods; (b) promote adequate nutrition and feeding practices in schools; and (c) provide indicators for monitoring and evaluating school feeding programs in Uganda. The guidelines focus on 11 major areas: school gardening and local food production, food procurement and transportation, food storage and preservation in schools, food hygiene, school food preparation and serving, nutrition and care, nutrition education and awareness promotion, vulnerable schoolchildren, school kitchens, food poisoning, and packed food. Although the guidelines are considered exhaustive, they are silent about the various school feeding options that schools may consider adopting and hence may not propel action at the school level without concrete guidance on the critical issue of how the food to be eaten at school could be provided. Addressing this gap is thus necessary to enable finalizing and disseminating these guidelines.

Food is a basic human right. Uganda subscribes to the Universal Declaration of Human Rights of 1948 and the UN Convention on the Rights of the Child of 1990. Article 25 of the Universal Declaration clearly describes food as one of the basic requirements to which everyone has a right, in addition to clothing, housing, and medical and other necessary social services. Article 26 asserts everyone's right to education, which shall be free, at least in the elementary and fundamental stages. Article 28 reaffirms this right and enjoins state parties to ensure availability and accessibility of different forms of secondary education, including general and vocational, and to take measures to ensure regular school attendance and to reduce dropout rates. Uganda has been able to fulfill the right to education through ongoing universal education programs at the primary and postprimary (lower-secondary and equivalent vocational education grades) education levels. School feeding is one of the strategies that are important in ensuring that the desired standards (just described) are met.

Increasing access to quality social services, enhancing human capital development, and promoting sustainable population and the use of environmental and natural resources are some of the strategic objectives of the National Development Plan (NDP) 2010/11 to 2014/15. School feeding issues feature in a number of NDP themes, which authenticates its relevance to national development. Within the population theme, promotion of school feeding programs to reduce hunger in school for improved nutritional status and school performance of children is one of the interventions that one hopes will be undertaken. Complementary to this goal is the revitalization of public health education about appropriate feeding, nutrition, and health, all of which have direct bearing on the focus of this analysis.

Building community and institutional capacity for management of malnutrition through nutrition education and then supporting institutional feeding are additional strategies that are relevant to the NDP's health theme. Mobilization of communities to participate in school activities is another area highlighted under the education theme within the strategic objective of improving effectiveness and efficiency of primary education. Similarly, the social development theme identifies the need to ensure effective community mobilization and participation in development initiatives with an aim of improving functionality of and accessibility to quality social services, including education. Because of its multisectoral nature, implementation of the NDP is the responsibility of the respective sector ministries under the coordination of Prime Minister's Office.

The Education (Pre-Primary, Primary, and Post-Primary) Act of 2008[1] clarifies the responsibilities of stakeholders in education and training. Provision of food and participation in community activities that support education are some of the key responsibilities of parents and guardians under the universal education programs. Foundation bodies are also mandated to mobilize resources for education purposes. The act further presents articles related to the prohibition of charges for education under the Universal Primary Education (UPE) and Uganda Post-Primary Education and Training (UPPET) programs. Specifically, article 9(1) states: "No person or agency shall levy or order another person to levy any charge for purposes of education in any primary or postprimary institution implementing UPE or UPPET program." Article 9(2) goes further to say: "The provisions of subsection 9(1) shall not be construed to deter the management of any school or institution implementing UPE or UPPET program from collecting or receiving voluntary contributions or payments from parents and well wishers to contain a state of emergency or any urgent matter concerning the school." Article 9(3) clarifies article 9(2) by stating: "No pupil or student shall be sent away from a school or an institution or denied access to education for failure to pay any contribution referred to under subsection 9(2)." Article 9(4) concludes: "A person who contravenes subsections (1), (2), and (3) commits an offence and is liable on conviction to a fine not exceeding fifty currency points or imprisonment not exceeding twelve months or both." Article 15 (2c) mandates head teachers to charge for midday meals in city and municipal council schools; in article 15(5), the provision is extended to all urban councils so they may charge for midday meals as determined by the management committees in consultation with district councils. Although these provisions are silent about rural schools, article

15(6) states that taking midday meals at school and payment for such meals shall be voluntary, and no pupil shall be excluded from school for nonpayment or for not taking food to school. This provision seems to embrace both rural and urban schools although rural schools have not exploited it. Limiting payment of lunch fees to only urban schools is unjustified.

The following sector policies have a bearing on school feeding in Uganda:

- The draft School Health Policy of 2008 is aimed at attaining a healthy school community and environment to contribute to the achievement of optimal education performance, socioeconomic well-being, and national development. One of its specific policy objectives is promoting the provision of nutrition and school feeding services, as well as strengthening and enforcing the implementation of complementary health-related policies and interventions in educational institutions, including those stipulated in the Minimum Health Care Package. The draft policy reaffirms that attaining education as a fundamental human right requires good health and nutrition, and it recognizes schools as the most efficient and effective means of reaching large proportions of the population. The draft policy indicates that the overall responsibility of school health will be led by the Ministry of Education and Sports and identifies the Ministry of Health as a key player. Institutional structures to be established as identified in the draft policy include the multisectoral National School Health Steering Committee and the National School Health Coordination Unit. Lower-level organs include District School Health Committees, Subcounty School Health Committees, and School Health Committees. The draft plan is also supported by a draft School Health Strategic Plan 2010–15, which will be implemented as soon as the policy is passed and resources are earmarked in the budget. The policy's integration of school feeding within the broader school health perspectives is a welcomed move.

- The Food and Nutrition Policy aims at improving food security, improving nutritional status, and increasing income through multisectoral and interdisciplinary interventions. The policy also sets a firm basis for improving school feeding. The policy's specific objectives include (a) ensuring availability, accessibility, and affordability of food in the quantities and qualities sufficient to satisfy the dietary needs of individuals; (b) promoting good nutrition of the population; (c) incorporating food and nutrition issues in all development plans; (d) ensuring that nutrition education and training is provided to improve knowledge and attitudes for behavioral change; (e) monitoring the food and nutrition situation of the country; (f) advocating for food and nutrition; (g) promoting policy, laws, and standards for food security and nutrition; and (h) ensuring a healthy environment and good sanitation for the entire food chain. These objectives are highly relevant in promoting nutrition of children, especially if schools are used as implementation anchors for this policy. However, nutrition promotion and monitoring are not undertaken in schools. The policy also proposes establishment of the Uganda Food and Nutrition Council as a key promotional organ of such initiatives, but it has not yet been implemented.

- The decentralization policy devolves primary education service delivery to district local governments, which indicates their central role in ensuring that school management teams and parents or guardians execute their functions for efficient and effective education service delivery.

Strategic plans such as the National Strategic Plan for Orphans and Other Vulnerable Children (2004) highlight school feeding in their list of priorities. The five-year plan developed by the Ministry of Gender, Labour, and Social Development is grounded on the belief that investment in social development provides opportunities to tackle imbalances and inequities within society. In recognition of the presence of vulnerable population categories in the country that may need special protection, the plan seeks to secure an adequate liveli-hood within the equity-led growth policies of the government of Uganda. The plan reaffirms education as a fundamental right for every child and as a means through which targeting of the most vulnerable can be enhanced, and it strives to promote essential social sector links by targeting retention at school of vulner-able children at risk of dropping out or those who have recently dropped out. Key interventions in the plan include short-term community-based programs such as school feeding. The delayed start-up of these initiatives has been attrib-uted to financial constraints.

Some strategies and programs have been put in place by different sectors, in particular the Ministry of Health, in an attempt to improve the health and nutrition status of children, but these have not yet extended to schools. They include the following programs:

- Micronutrient supplementation programs that distribute iron and vitamin A supplements to communities twice a year under the Child Days program.
- The Micronutrient Strategies and Technology program, which has facilitated food fortification of maize (mixing the food with micronutrients such as iron, zinc, calcium, and B vitamins). The program targets industries that supply boarding and private schools, which does not benefit students of government day primary and secondary schools, most of whom do not receive meals at school. Those that do rely heavily on local food producers.
- Deworming during the national Child Days. Mass deworming during Child Days targets children six years of age and younger and is not extended to those in school. Schoolchildren between 6 and 15 years of age are known to carry the greatest burden of worms. For the past years, it was estimated that 50 percent of all school-age children might be infected with worms. However, Uganda has no good examples of mass deworming school programs. Current deworming programs under the Child Days Plus program are at community level although hosted at schools in some settings.

Note

1. Act 13, Supplement No. 8, the Education (Pre-Primary, Primary, and Post-Primary) Act of 2008.

CHAPTER 3

Community-Led School Feeding Practices

The World Food Programme (WFP) has promoted and supported school feeding in Uganda through geographical targeting of the most vulnerable with a great focus on the conflict areas of northern Uganda. Following the launch of the Peace, Recovery, and Development Plan for Northern Uganda, the school feeding program for the northern region was closed. Since 2008, the WFP school feeding program has been running only in the food-insecure Karamoja region districts. In all other districts, feeding of children is the mandate of the parents, as articulated in the Universal Primary Education (UPE) policy and the Education Act of 2008. This chapter provides highlights of the ongoing school-based initiatives, including operational challenges and strengths. Of note, the survey was exploratory in nature and focused on understanding the evolution and implementation of modalities of the various community-led school feeding options, *not* the impact of those initiatives on learning outcomes. Where appropriate, highlights from the 2009/10 Uganda National Household Survey (UNHS) and Uganda National Panel Survey, as well as the Quality Enhancement Initiative (QEI) survey have been provided.

Home-Packed Food for Consumption by Pupils at School

A home-packed meal for learners is the government's most promoted option and the only recommended school feeding model for rural schools. It involves pupils carrying packed food from home for consumption at school during the midmorning break (especially for lower-primary learners who attend half-day) or at lunch time for upper-primary learners who spend the full day at school. In districts such as Kibaale, schools adhere strictly to this modality. In the central and eastern regions, it is one of the options used by school pupils, whereas in the northern region it is the least desired option for sociocultural reasons.

Results from the QEI baseline survey of 2009 (figure 3.1) indicate that despite carrying a home-packed meal being the most promoted practice, its uptake is still low and only moderately reported in Kyenjojo (40 percent) and Lyantonde (38 percent) districts, followed by Buliisa (22 percent). The low uptake signals

Figure 3.1 Percentage of Pupils Who Carry Their Own Lunch to School by District, QEI Uganda 2009

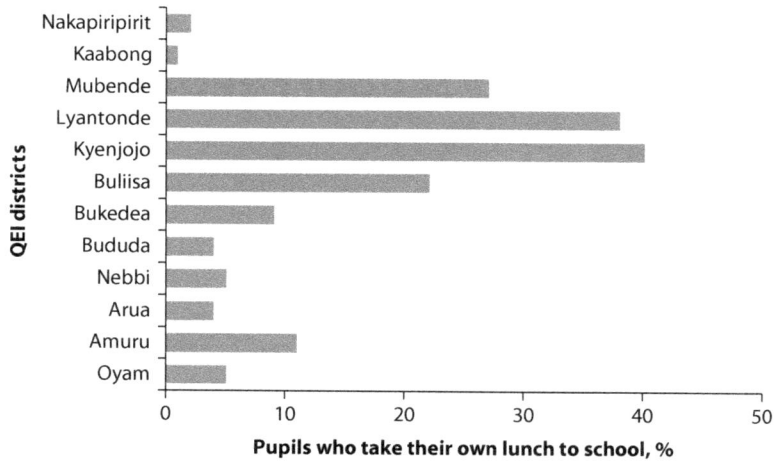

Source: Data from Quality Enhancement Initiative Baseline Survey, Uganda.

underlying challenges to its implementation by parents and raises concerns about what other options parents and schools need to consider so everyone can ensure that pupils are fed at school for effective learning. Nevertheless, the survey team undertook in-depth observations in schools with relatively high uptake levels, and the findings indicate that successful implementation of this feeding option depends largely on a number of factors that include the following:

- *Sustained community mobilization and sensitization by School Management Committees (SMCs) and political leadership using various communication channels.* In Kibaale district where this modality is reported to be relatively more successful, district officials and head teachers of sampled schools attributed that success largely to (a) the sustained community mobilization drive spearheaded by the district authorities and (b) the heavy involvement of SMCs in ensuring parental compliance. Responses from key informants (district officials and head teachers of sampled schools) included the following:
  - "The district council prioritizes school feeding, and local leaders encourage parents to feed their children at school wherever they get an opportunity in churches, mosques, and other public functions."
  - "There are many messages on the importance of school feeding that are disseminated on our local radio."
  - "We have run a school feeding campaign on the local radio for the past two years, and parents are now fully aware of the importance of school feeding, but there are many challenges."
- *Type of food available.* Some food types were reported to be easier to pack than others. Cereals (maize, rice) and tubers such as cassava, sweet potatoes, and Irish potatoes were reported to be easier to pack because they can be eaten

cold and without sauce. Other food types such as matooke or millet bread (*atapa*, *karo*) and cassava bread and maize meal, which are the most common staple foods in Uganda, were reported to be culturally ineligible for packing because they are served hot and eaten with sauce. The survey team, however, noted that fruits were not seen pupils' packs despite their being not only easy to pack but also more available in the communities.

- *School-level norms that support parental adherence.* Integration of requirements such as food containers on the school admission list, endorsed and signed consent forms by the parents to enforce their commitment to the practice, and daily morning checks by class teachers to ensure all pupils have complied with the packed-food requirements were identified as important school management practices that are essential for sustained parental adherence to this modality.

- *Parental commitment.* Food packing is a daily and routine event, thus its continuity is highly dependent on parental commitment, as indicated in the statements from the pupils' focus groups in Kibaale district:
  - "My mother ensures she has something to put in my food container before going to bed every day."
  - "At my home, my parents always check our containers before we go to school, and we always have to take them back home after school because without them, we would have nothing to use for the following day and would also not be allowed in school."

- *Food availability at the household level.* Either leftover food at supper that children can carry to school the following day (implying a surplus at household level), or food that can easily be prepared with ease in the morning, or quick dry snacks and fruits that can be easily packed by learners are required. A combination of these could be used. Lack of food was cited in all focus groups as the major reason for parental failure to pack food for their children. For example, some parents said:
  - "We do not have leftover food in our homes for children to take to school."
  - "We do not have food in this area because of the long dry spells that we have had and hence cannot pack anything for children."

- *Family size.* Parents reported that food packing is easier for parents with few children compared to those with many, because the latter calls for more food and time requirements than the former. Uganda's total fertility rate stands at about 6.7 children per woman. Using the life cycle model, one can estimate that approximately 60 percent of families on average have three or four children attending primary school.

The survey team examined samples of packed food to establish food preparation and packing practices. They made the following observations: (a) most packed food for pupils is prepared in the evening as part of the family supper, implying that it stays for a long time before it is eaten, increasing chances of food poisoning; (b) no food preservation was observed, and most food is either steamed or boiled and hence likely to go bad easily if not well handled; and (c) food packaging materials varied from plastic food containers to polythene bags. The use of banana leaves and fibers was seen in some remote rural schools, as well as materials with potential health risks such as containers for detergents.

Handling of food packs at school and operational modalities. Modes of storing food packs for learners varied from school to school. Some schools had designated areas for keeping pupils' packed food, which included identified corners with a table or rack at the back of classrooms and in some instances lockable small rooms, some of which had shelves, as was the case in some of the schools in Kibaale district. In other schools without designated areas, food packs or containers could be found everywhere, including window sills, on top of

Management of Packed Meals in Schools

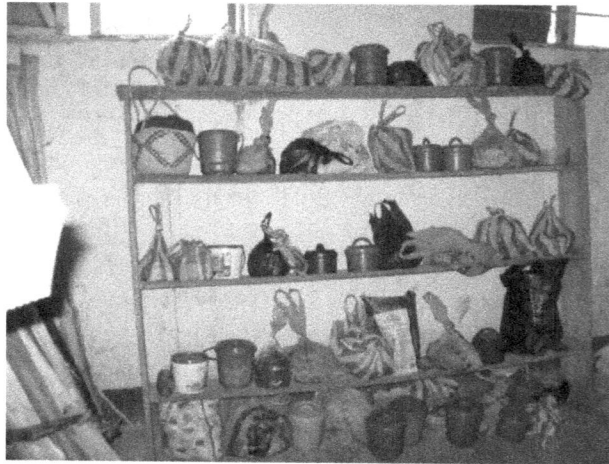

Source: © Mr. Charles Lwanga Bunjo

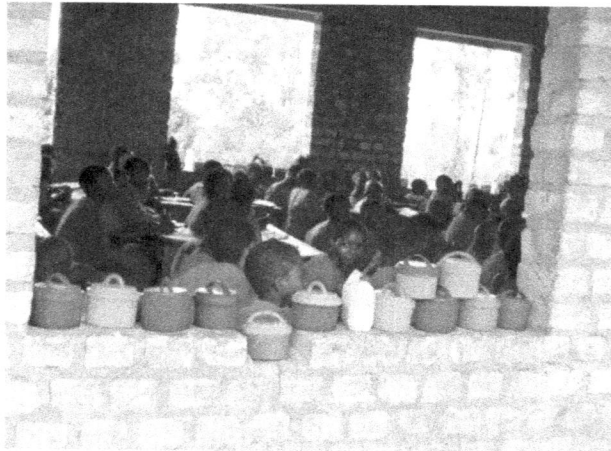

Source: © Mr. Charles Lwanga Bunjo

Management of Packed Meals in Schools *(continued)*

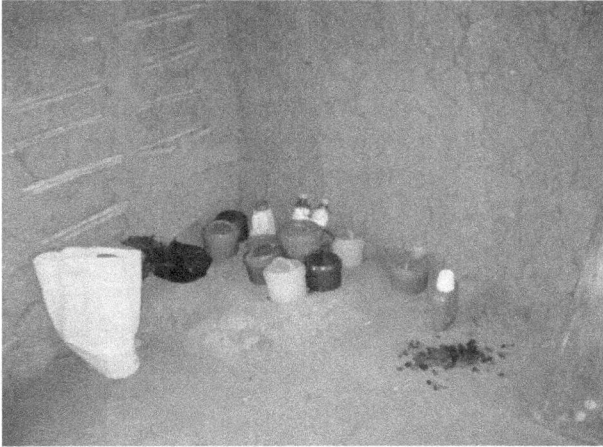

Source: © Mr. Charles Lwanga Bunjo

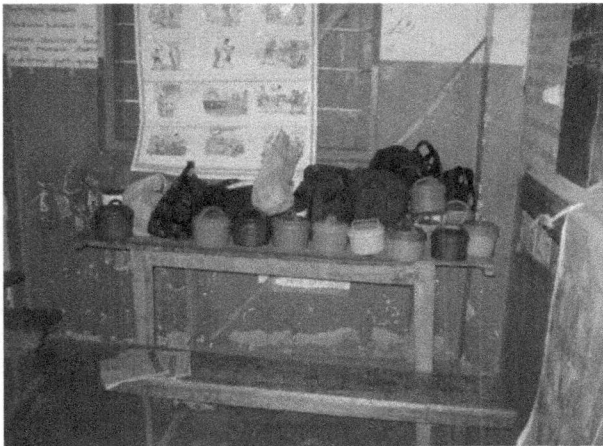

Source: © Mr. Charles Lwanga Bunjo

learners' desks, or even on the floors, thus creating a rather untidy classroom environment compounded by the big class sizes. Teacher supervision of learners when they picked up their food containers was observed in some schools.

Eating schedules observed to vary by grade. Grade 1 and 2 learners would eat their packed meals during the midmorning break, whereas learners of other grades would eat at midday. Some learners in the latter category would eat half their meal at midmorning and reserve the rest for the lunch meal, with implications on food-handling practices and likely risks, especially where hygienic practices are not well instituted.

Schools with no designated eating places. Pupils will eat at convenient places in the school compound as found appropriate. These places include tree-shaded areas, classrooms, and verandahs. Hand-washing facilities were observed in very few schools. The facilities should enable children to wash their hands before and after meals, including washing their containers after meals. However, this cleanup step was not the case in a good number of observed schools, reflecting the poor hygiene standards in schools and the unavailability of opportunities for learners to practice regularly promoted health messages such as "washing hands before and after meals" in a transformative setting such as a school.

An analysis of strengths, weaknesses, opportunities, and threats (SWOT) generated the following in regard to home-packed meals (see table 3.1). See box 3.1 for more about home-packed meals.

Table 3.1 SWOT Analysis of Home-Packed Meals

Strengths and opportunities	Weaknesses and threats

• Packed meals are relatively less exclusionary, especially in situations where the school administration is involved in ensuring adherence.
• Food packing is an older practice and easier to promote.
• No time is lost in its management, and the burden lies largely with the parents because packs are child specific.
• A packed meal ensures full engagement of parents and guardians in the well-being of children by virtue of its regular nature.
• It promotes prudence regarding food security issues at the household level among responsible parents.
	• Packing a meal is daily and routine in nature and hence imposes substantial time constraints at the household level.
	• A packed meal is more acceptable to lower-grade pupils than to those in upper grades whose food requirements are more than for the former. For example, some pupils in the focus groups stated:
	  - "That method is outdated and grown-up children and boys cannot carry food packs."
	  - "The food provided in the container is too little and is not enough for P5–P7 pupils."
	  - "Food containers are for girls not boys who need to eat much more."
	• Children from households without food or packing facilities are likely to be excluded.
	• Adherence is not regular among learners because food packing is highly dependent on a number of factors including (a) food type and availability at the household level and (b) degree of parental commitment and involvement.
	• Teachers do not have to cater the children's food under this arrangement.
	• School setting of standards is a challenge because of the diverse nature of households and welfare levels. In some instances, children were reported to have brought alcoholic drinks such as *Omuramba* or *Kwete* as reported in Kabale district, or symbolic items (for example, raw fruits or very little amounts of food were cited) that are not suitable or even sufficient to constitute a meal.
	• Food hygiene is difficult to ensure. Food is prepared overnight, and unpreserved food is mostly stored at room temperature, increasing chances of getting spoilage with resultant food poisoning.
	• Fear of poisoning pupils through food packs is rampant in some areas, especially the West Nile region. Some head teachers and parents talked to in Maracha district stated:
	  - "We cannot pack food for our children because it would make them easy targets by our enemies."
	  - "Individual packs for children are very dangerous in our community, and head teachers would be held responsible for anything that happens to the children."
	• Improper food packaging and storage facilities at the school level, coupled with lack of appropriate containers for children, constrain effective implementation of this modality.
	• Households with large families have difficulty implementing this modality.

Source: World Bank data.

Box 3.1

Home-Packed Meals for Pupils in St. Elizabeth Bujuni Primary School, Kibaale District

St. Elizabeth Bujuni Primary School in Kibaale is a Catholic school started in 1926 by the White Fathers. With an enrollment of 718 pupils (44 percent girls), it is one of the schools that has successfully implemented the home-packed meals school feeding option since its inception. Coverage was estimated at 98 percent, and it is the only method of school feeding that is used in the school.

The high compliance level was attributed to the following: A food container is one of the items a learner should have in addition to a school uniform and scholastic materials. When parents or guardians sign a commitment form at the children's admission to school, they pledge to provide packed food to their children. Parents reaffirm this commitment every year.

Daily morning checks are undertaken by all class teachers to ensure all the children have packed meals as they enter classrooms.

Each classroom has a special corner or table where food is kept until midmorning break and lunchtime. Some pupils eat part of their food at the midmorning break, and the other part is taken at lunchtime.

Common foods packed include cassava, Irish potatoes, matooke, and beans. Those who can afford it add avocado, which is a very common fruit in this area and also serves as a sauce.

Although the school has a borehole, pupils are advised to carry their drinking water from home.

Challenges identified by the school administration include eating cold or leftover food by the pupils with likely negative consequences on food hygiene standards; unsealable or inappropriate containers, in some instances leading to food spillage in the classrooms; and drought periods during which household food security is low, resulting in higher than usual default rates.

Regular radio messages by the district officials reinforce the school and parental actions toward this initiative.

Source: World Bank data.

Preparation and Provision of Hot Meals to Pupils at School

Preparation and provision of hot meals to pupils at school is another practice that prevails in schools outside the WFP areas of Karamoja but to a much lesser degree. In this modality, hot meals are prepared at school in accordance with agreements between the parents and the school administration. Initiation of this practice involves discussions among the parents through the SMC. Information on agreed modalities is communicated to parents through existing institutions, including the local council meetings and prayer sessions, school notice boards, and school open days (whenever they are held).

Of importance is that this modality is considered illegal in rural schools by all national and district officials talked to, and getting information on practicing schools was no mean feat. However, the 2008 Education Act, article 15(5), provides room for schools to engage parents in this regard as earlier indicated; therefore, the few practicing schools should be protected under this provision.

The research findings indicate that implementation of this school feeding option is enabled by in-kind food contributions by parents, cash contributions toward school meals, and food harvests from the school gardens. Each of these modalities has its unique characteristics as indicated in the following subsections.

In-Kind Food Contributions by Parents to Schools

This practice is most common in rural parts of Uganda, especially the grain and cereal-growing regions.

- The food contributions are made by school terms (three times a year), but leftover food from one term is carried over to the next term.
- The food quantity contributed per child is determined by the SMC in consultation with the Parents and Teachers Association (PTA) Executive Committee. It also depends on the type of food served (solid meals or semisolid such as porridge) and the number of meals a child has at school (midmorning especially for P1–P2, lunch, or both), as also indicated in table 3.2.

The survey observed that food contributions (type and quantity) vary from school to school, depending on food grown in the area (beans; maize, especially in the eastern, western, and northern regions; millet and sorghum, mostly in the west and parts of the north) and type of meal to be prepared by the school.

Table 3.2 Type of Contributions Made, by Observed School and District, Uganda 2011

District	Primary school	Type of meal	Contributions per child per term		
			Maize (kgs)	Bean (kgs)	Cash[a] (U Sh)
Busia	Madibira	Solid meal	15	7.5	2,500
		Porridge	5	n.a.	2,500
	Mukwanya	Solid meal	10	5	1,500
		Porridge	5	n.a.	1,000
Bukedea	Kotolut	Solid meal	7.5	2.5	2,000
	Bukedea	Solid meal	8	4	2,000
Maracha	Ambekua	Solid meal	30[b]	5	10,000
	Bura	Solid meal	25[b]	5	5,000
Isingiro	Ntungu Mixed	Solid meal	[c]	5	2,500
Amolatar	Amolatar	Solid meal	15	10	3,000
	Kataleba	Porridge	10	n.a.	500

Source: World Bank data.

Note: n.a. = not applicable.

a. Cash contributions are used to pay cooks, to buy firewood and salt, and to grind maize.

b. Cassava flour.

c. Millennium Village Project supplies maize flour.

Table 3.2 captures some of the findings. Maize and beans were the most common foods contributed by parents toward their children's hot meal at school, although cassava was also contributed in kind in Maracha district. Solid meals fetch higher food quantities than do the semisolid meals (hot maize or millet porridge), and the quantities varied from one school to another even within the same district. For example, pupils of Mudibira Primary School in Busia district were contributing 15 kilograms of maize or corn for a solid meal compared to 10 kilograms for those in Mukwanya Primary School. Across districts surveyed, Bukedea district registered the lowest contribution toward a solid meal (7.5 kilograms in Kotolut Primary School). Similarly, quantities contributed toward semisolid meals (porridge) varied, ranging from a low of 5 kilograms of maize per pupil in Busia district to a high of 10 kilograms in Amolator district. In addition, bean contributions varied from 2.5 kilograms in Bukedea to 10 kilograms in Amolator district. Harmonization of quantity consumed per child thus emerges as an issue that deserves consideration, especially within districts.

In-kind contributions are not sufficient to earn children a meal. Additional cash payments are made to facilitate grain processing or milling and food preparation processes, which include purchasing firewood, paying cooks' wages, and buying water (reported in schools without safe water sources). As is the case with food quantities, complementary cash contributions toward a solid meal varied from a low of U Sh 1,500 in Mukwanya Primary School of Busia district to a high of U Sh 10,000 in Ambekua Primary School of Maracha district. However, the complementary cash contribution toward semisolid meals varied narrowly from a low of U Sh 500 in Kataleba Primary School of Amolator district to U Sh 2,500 in Madibira Primary School of Busia district. Processing and labor costs are expected to vary from one location to another, which may largely explain the variations in the cash contributions that complement the in-kind food contributions. Harmonization of those costs may not be easy even within districts and calls for better understanding of the local markets, including availability of certain services such as milling within reasonable reach of schools.

In some schools visited, food processing is the responsibility of the food committee (which comprises participating parents, SMC representatives, teachers, and pupils—the last mostly welfare prefects). All processing is done in small quantities that are sufficient to last a week to avoid contamination and waste, and it uses local transportation and processing services.

The survey also probed the extent to which parents adhered to this feeding option. All head teachers who were talked to reported irregularity in contributions, which they attributed largely to seasonal factors. In-kind food contributions were reported to be most regular during harvest seasons (see also box 3.2). However, head teachers noted that in dry and low-yield seasons, parental adherence to their food commitments toward schools was very low, which is a great risk to the sustainability of this school feeding option. Enforcement was reported to be constrained by the covert manner in which this modality is practiced at

Box 3.2

In-Kind Food Contributions in Kotolut Primary School, Bukedea District

Kotolut Primary School is a rural school in Bukedea district, 17 kilometers from the district headquarters. It is one of the few schools practicing the in-kind food contribution scheme for school feeding.

Parents voluntarily contribute 7.5 kilograms of maize and 2.5 kilograms of beans. An additional U Sh 2,000 per child per term is paid to facilitate grinding of maize, paying the cooks, and buying salt.

By the time of the survey, 150 of the 700 pupils (21.4 percent) were participating in the scheme.

The school plans to request parents to allocate home gardens to their children to enable them to grow their own food, from which they would bring part to the school. This strategy would increase participation in the scheme and would enhance household food security.

Source: World Bank data.

school level. Other challenges cited include failure to estimate the actual food requirements per child, which often leads to underestimation of food contributions required. Some of the responses from head teachers that reflect those issues include the following:

- "The food quantity contributed per child is just an estimate, but we are not sure of the exact amounts that should be contributed."
- "Some parents do not fulfill their commitments, and we fear reminding them because they may report to political leaders at the district."
- "In some instances, the food contributed runs out before the term ends, and it's hard to ask parents for more food."

Cash Contributions for Meals by Parents to Schools

Voluntary contribution of an agreed sum of money by parents that is used by the school administration to purchase food items is another school feeding practice observed in the sampled schools and was reported to be the most common and legally practiced modality in urban and peri-urban areas. Where this modality was observed (with the exception of Kampala schools), schools used it as a voluntary but special consideration for the candidate classes (Primary 7 and in a few instances Primary 6) in a bid to alleviate the short-term hunger that was likely to affect students' concentration and lead to anticipated poor performance—especially in the final examinations. Teachers in some of the practicing schools are allowed to contribute toward their meals although the charge was found to be higher than that paid by pupils.

Table 3.3 Cash Contributions for Hot Meals, by School, and Estimated Cost for DEOs and Head Teachers

District	School	Type of meal	Actual cash contribution (U Sh)	Estimated cost of feeding by DEO/DIS (U Sh)	Estimated cost by head teachers (U Sh)
Kabale	Kabale	Solid meal	25,000	30,000	33,000
	Rwere	Porridge[a]	Funded	5,000	3,000
Kampala	Kasubi	Solid meal	20,000	30,000	30,000
		Porridge	15,000	20,000	20,000
	Makerere	Solid meal	20,500	20,000	25,000
		Porridge	15,500	15,000	20,000
Kayunga	Bishop Brown	Solid meal	25,000	30,000	30,000
		Porridge	5,000	10,000	10,000
	Bulawula	Porridge	School-grown maize	10,000	8,000
Mpigi	Kibuuka Memorial	Solid meal[b]	Funded	20,000	25,000
		Porridge	5,500	5,000	6,000
	Muduuma	Porridge	8,000	5,000	10,000

Source: World Bank data.
Note: DEO = District Education Officer, DIS = District Inspector of Schools.
a. Funded externally by Lady Catherine through the diocese of Kigezi.
b. Funded by CHISOM (Child Support Organisation Mpigi).

The findings on amounts contributed in selected schools are captured in table 3.3. Following are some of the highlights:

- The amount of money contributed per child per term varied from school to school but was based on considerations of average food prices within the school communities. The amount was agreed among the SMC, the representatives of parents, and the school administration before communication to willing parents. This amount ranged from U Sh 5,000 to U Sh 8,000 for the semisolid meal and from U Sh 15,000 to U Sh 25,000 for a solid meal.
- The mode of payment also varied with locality. For Kampala schools, for example, the funds are deposited to school accounts in commercial banks, and payment slips are presented to schools, whereas in other areas, parents deposit the cash contributions at schools. Monthly installments were the most commonly reported by schools because of the low income levels of most parents, but that method poses a challenge to record management at the school level. Transparency has to be maintained, however, to sustain the trust of participating parents.
- Food purchase was undertaken by the school administration. Schools visited have either a focal point officer or welfare teacher, along with the school bursar or deputy head teacher who are charged with this role. Some schools have food committees; for example, in one school the committee consisted of five persons (two women and three men). With or without committees, most schools have a designated focal person in charge of purchasing food items.

- Weekly food purchases were reported, and the reasons for this schedule ranged from lack of adequate storage space to the need to avoid food waste. This timing has implications for school-level planning and issues related to regular cash purchases. Responses included the following:
  - "We cannot buy more than what is needed in a week because we do not have enough space to keep it."
  - "Weekly food purchases ease our planning."
  - "It is hard to keep processed maize flour for long in our environment. It would go bad."
- Clear procurement systems were reported only in Kampala schools, but other observed schools reported using existing community markets without clear systems on how this is done. Buying from local markets is advantageous in providing business for the local population and promoting the local economies.

Despite the small number of participating pupils, the school administrations reported high default rates in this modality because it is highly dependent on parental willingness and ability to pay, it is voluntary, and (most important) it is covertly practiced so that noncompliance cannot be punished. The ever-increasing food prices were also noted as a major hindrance to realistic cost estimation by schools. In some instances, schools reported requesting that participating parents pay more money midterm after the realization that the initially contributed funds were insufficient. For example, one of the head teachers reported: "The price of maize has been increasing almost every fortnight and the money that was contributed got finished a month before the term ended, which we had not anticipated."

Another teacher mentioned: "Some parents default midway through the term, and when we remind them, they threaten to report the school management to the Resident District Commissioner." Nevertheless, key informants interviewed at the schools and the districts as well as parents felt this modality would be the most preferred if the government would agree to it for all schools rather than only for urban schools. Consensus existed that parents would be more willing to make cash contributions toward their children's meals at school as is done in urban schools if it is officially approved by government.

Food Harvested from School Gardens

Some schools, especially in the rural areas, have school gardens where food is grown and harvested for consumption at the school level. Availability of school gardens of ample size is a very rare occurrence in densely populated areas and at times is complicated by land ownership norms. The following findings are from some of the sample schools with school gardens (see also box 3.3).

- Food was grown by pupils during agriculture lessons.
- Farm land size was between five and seven acres.
- Pupils contribute seeds—mainly corn and beans.

Box 3.3

School Gardening for School Feeding in Bulawula Primary School, Kayunga District

Bulawula Primary School is a rural school located in Kayunga district, 20 kilometers from the district headquarters, and is one of the schools in the district that provide food to learners from the school garden.

The school garden covers five acres and is cultivated by students (an estimated two days per term was reported). The first day is when pupils clear the land and plant the maize. The second day when they work in the garden is for weeding. On each of the days, learners spend only 30 minutes in the garden, and this time is scheduled.

With a good yield, the school harvests 20 bags of 100 kilograms each, totaling 2,000 kilograms of maize. The produce is used as follows:

- 12 bags (1,200 kilograms) for feeding pupils
- 3 bags (300 kilograms) for feeding the teachers
- 5 bags (500 kilograms) sold to cover grinding, paying the cooks, and renovating the school.

With low yields, probably caused by inadequate rains, pupils are not fed. Pupils contribute the seeds, and each pupil brings about one-quarter of a kilogram of maize seeds (which is measured with a standard plastic cup).

All other issues to do with the gardening are handled by the SMC and teachers.

Identified strengths are (a) enrollment increases during the school feeding time when the yield is good, and (b) the program increases children's interest in farming.

Identified challenges are (a) seasonality of the program, (b) weather changes that affect yields, and (c) destruction of crops by stray animals.

Source: World Bank data.

- Output varied by season, and feeding of pupils using this modality was also seasonal.
- All management issues were handled by the school administration and the SMC.

Lessons could also be drawn from the WFP School Gardens Project, which was implemented as an integral part of the concluded Food for Education Program in 2008. The project was a bid to facilitate a smooth transition of the schools and communities from WFP's central food provision to self-reliance. Under this initiative, sensitization of school management teams was undertaken, and support was extended to schools to clear 10 acres of land for crops. Parents who participated in the land clearing, weeding, and harvesting were given food items under the WFP's Food for Assets (FFA) program in exchange for their labor. Partnerships were also formed with civil society organizations such as SOCADIDO (the social development nongovernmental organization of the Catholic Church in the eastern region), which undertook distribution of inputs to schools. Those materials included seeds, potato vines, cassava cuttings, and initial setting up of gardens in some areas. Some schools formed committees responsible for school gardening (FFA or Food Management or School Agriculture Committees), while others selected appropriate but existing school committees to oversee this initiative. The food grown was either consumed by the schools or sold to purchase other critical inputs such as oxen and plows for sustainability purposes.

Challenges identified include negative parental attitudes in some communities, low response of some school management teams, sustainability of providing inputs to schools, lack of community awareness and skills to manage some crops, delays in providing incentives supplied through the FFA program that demoralized participating parents, and bad weather conditions such as floods and prolonged drought that affected crop yields. Okure Primary School in Soroti district was one of the success stories that could be captured from the WFP monitoring reports (see box 3.4).

Beneficiaries of Hot Meals. Beneficiaries of hot meals varied by school according to the arrangements between the SMCs and the school administration. Most commonly observed target groups at various schools included the following:

- Only those who cannot pack meals but who can pay the agreed sum of money were allowed to participate, irrespective of grade.
- Only Primary 7 pupils participated, which safeguarded them from disruptions to learning that were likely to affect end-of-cycle exam grades. (In some schools, the modality was mandatory for all Primary 7 pupils to avoid discrimination and to ensure that they were all well motivated throughout the year for better end-cycle grades.)
- The only pupils of grades 1 and 2 who participated were those whose parents decided that schools provides hot midmorning meals (porridge) to their children at school or a lunch meal for those who stay at school for the whole day, depending on parental preference.
- A combination of pupils from Primary 1 and grades 1 and 2 participated.

A look at the QEI data is important to get a rough assessment of how widespread this modality is based on the 12 QEI districts. Figures 3.2 and 3.3 indicate that the coverage of this school feeding mechanism is very low, especially when one looks at district specific data. Only the Karamoja region districts report moderate rates because of the WFP program (Kaabong has 67 percent and Nakapiripirit has 58 percent). Non-WFP districts that ranked next highest were the central region districts of Mubende (37 percent) and Lyantonde (20 percent). The practice was reported nonexistent in 7 of the 12 survey districts, largely because of the prohibition on parental contributions to schools under the UPE program.

Box 3.4

School Gardening for School Feeding in Okure Primary School Community, Soroti District, with Support from the WFP

Okure Community School's feeding initiative was undertaken with support from WFP's FFA project, which enabled the following:

- Clearing of 10 acres of land for crops to support the primary school by providing inputs and food items to participating parents through the WFP/FFA project
- Training with special focus on nutrition education
- Providing of inputs, which was undertaken by SOCADIDO of the Soroti district

The following table provides a summary of food quantities produced by the school with the inputs supplied:

Crop	Acreage in land	Quantity produced (kgs)
Cassava	3	2,172
Maize	2	520
Sweet potatoes	3	1,395
Beans	1	325
Onions	0.25	85
Tomatoes	0.25	79
Cabbage and eggplants	0.50	810
Totals	**10**	**5,386**

Reported benefits include increased enrollment, opportunity for parents to learn about food types and their nutritional importance to children, introduction of new food varieties to the community, access to balanced diets for schoolchildren during harvest seasons, and availability of food for children even when delays occurred in the provision of WFP rations to schools.

Challenges included unpredictability of yields caused by bad weather, stray animals (pigs, cattle, goats), negative attitudes by some parents, and inability to sustain provision of inputs and assets after the FFA program ended.

Source: WFP project reports, Uganda.

Food Preparation Modalities for Hot Meals. Food preparation modalities were observed in the sample schools, and the following key features were identified:

- Cooking of food is undertaken in either temporary or makeshift kitchens or cooking spaces, including under shady tree. This setting has implications for food quality and handling aspects, thus creating potential health hazards.

Figure 3.2 Percentage of Primary School Who Get Lunch at School; QEI Baseline, Uganda 2009/10

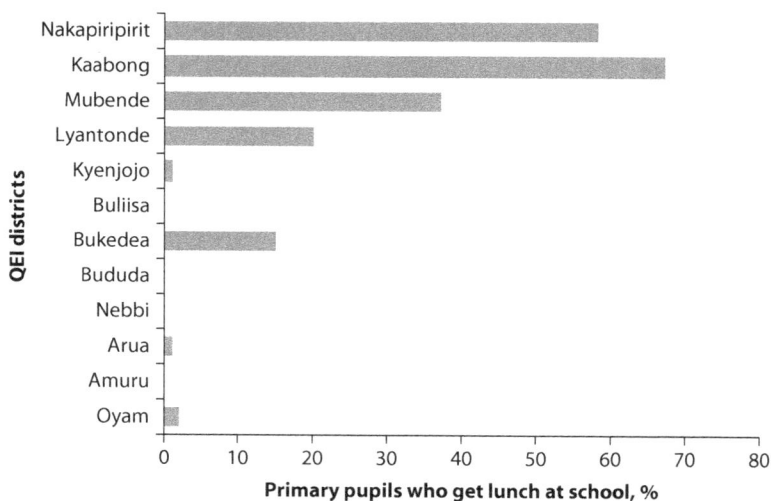

Source: Data from Quality Enhancement Initiative Baseline Survey, Uganda.

Figure 3.3 Percentage of Primary School that Provide Lunch at School; UNPS, 2009/10

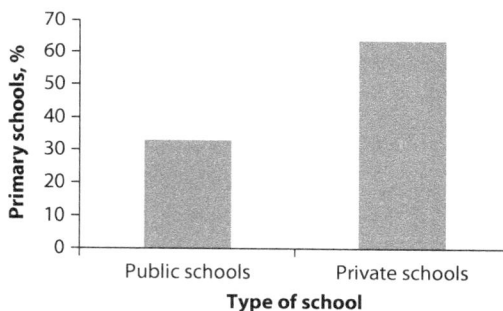

Source: Data from the Uganda Bureau of Statistics.

- Firewood was the main source of fuel used. Use of energy-saving stoves was observed only in schools where external support was being provided (for example, in WFP-supported districts, Isingiro Millennium Development Village project schools, and other schools that had accessed some external support beyond parental contributions).
- Nutritional aspects were not considered. Sugar for the porridge; cooking oil; and fruits, greens, and vegetables were not provided in any of the non-WFP schools, which affects the caloric and protein content of the food.
- Standardization of the quantity prepared was more easily done under in-kind food contribution than in the cash contribution modality. The quantity and food menu prepared varied from one school to another according to the amount of money paid and the food types available in the locality or contributed by parents.

Serving of Food and Eating Places. The survey further revealed that in most schools, the cooks serve the food. However, participation of student leaders such

Pictures of School Cooking Shades and Kitchens in Schools

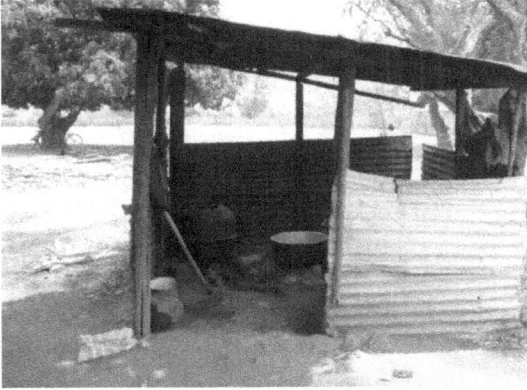

Source: © Mr. Charles Lwanga Bunjo

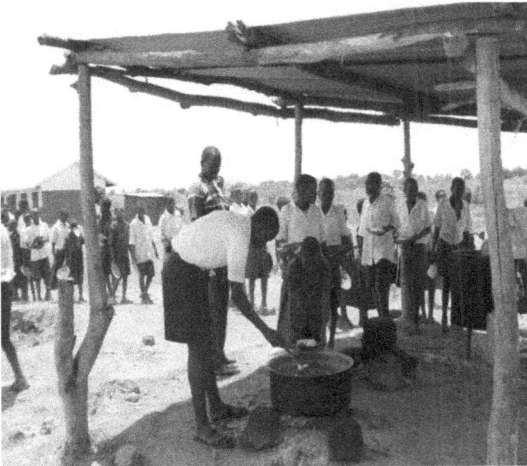

Source: © Mr. Charles Lwanga Bunjo

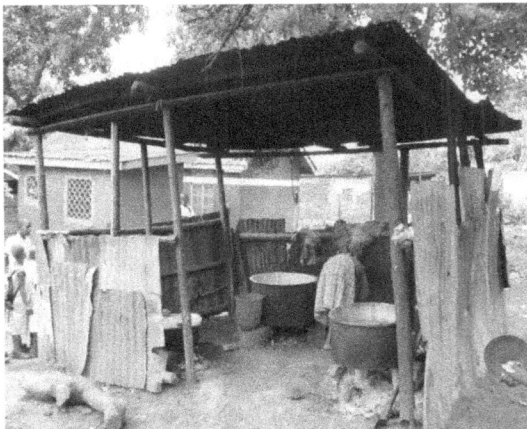

Source: © Mr. Charles Lwanga Bunjo

Pictures of School Cooking Shades and Kitchens in Schools *(continued)*

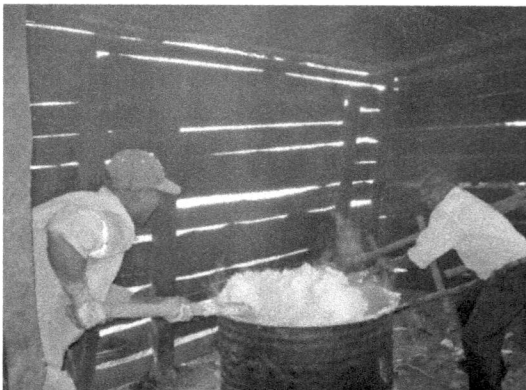

Source: © Mr. Charles Lwanga Bunjo

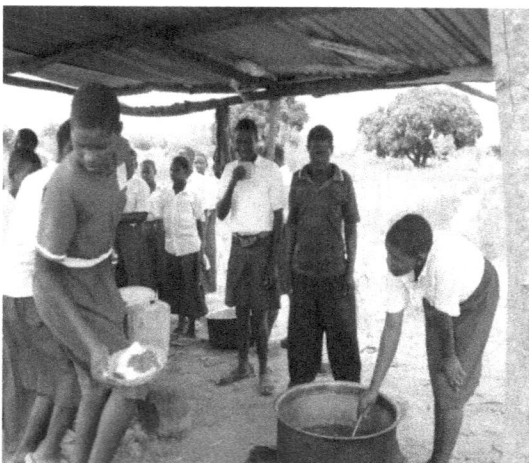

Source: © Mr. Charles Lwanga Bunjo

as prefects and teachers was observed in some schools. At food-serving times, parental and teacher involvement in monitoring was noted in some schools. Their participation enables the provision of the right food quantities to learners. It is also the time when eligible students are validated. Some schools had introduced meal cards to facilitate the daily validation process. Parental involvement enhances transparency and ownership, which are essential to the continuity of these schemes.

Food was served from the cooking points because of a lack of organized eating places or of shady areas similar to dining rooms in schools. Students bring their cups and plates from home.

Food serving is done in a number of ways, including by grade (lower grades are served before upper grades), by gender (separate points for boys and girls), or on a first-come, first-served basis, depending on the order in which classes with participating learners are released by teachers for the lunch break.

Pictures of How Hot Meals Are Served in Schools

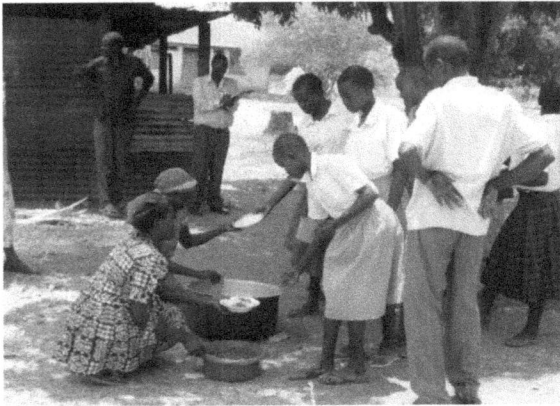

Source: © Mr. Charles Lwanga Bunjo

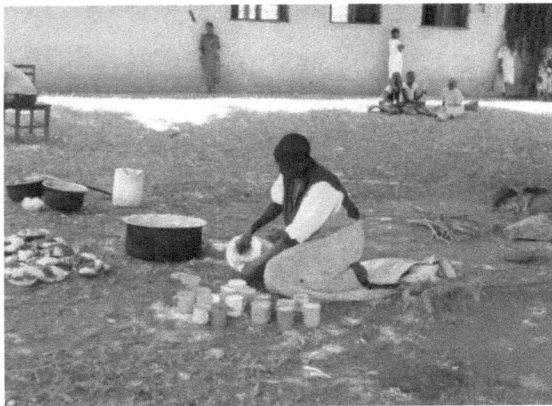

Source: © Mr. Charles Lwanga Bunjo

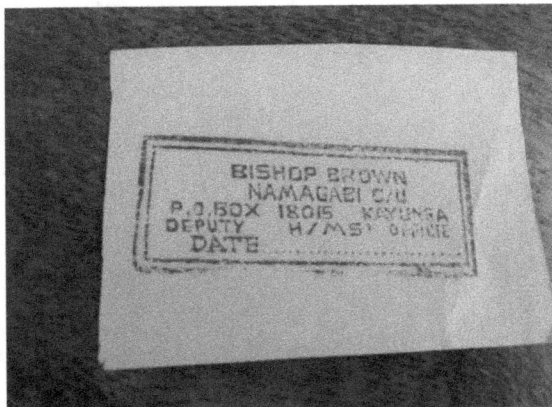

Source: © Mr. Charles Lwanga Bunjo

Pictures of How Hot Meals Are Served in Schools *(continued)*

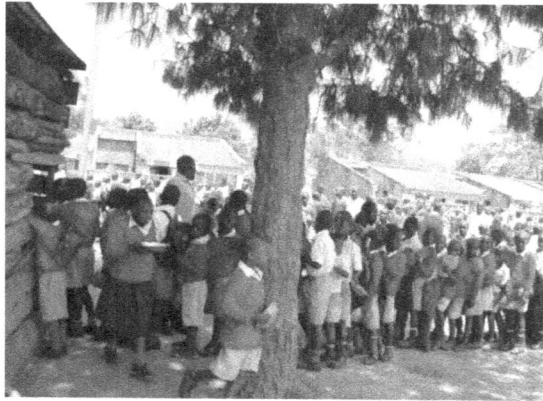

Source: © Mr. Charles Lwanga Bunjo

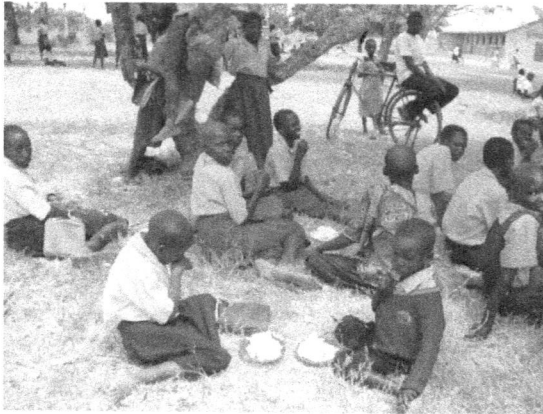

Source: © Mr. Charles Lwanga Bunjo

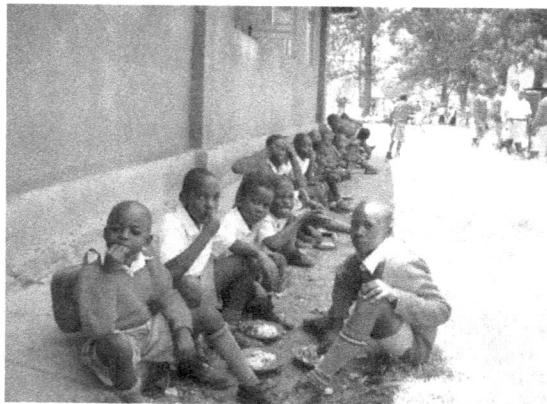

Source: © Mr. Charles Lwanga Bunjo

It is evident that hygienic practices not only in food preparation but also in food serving and eating by the learners need to be observed in the promotion of these modalities. The field team noted that washing hands before meals was largely not practiced in schools. This lack was attributed to the haphazard manner in which food is prepared and served. In addition, hand-washing water points are normally around school latrines, which are always distant from food preparation and serving areas. Identifying proper eating areas at respective schools would go a long way toward guiding school management teams about the need to equip such areas with necessary utilities, most importantly water.

A SWOT analysis was undertaken in regard to this modality, and the following was observed (see table 3.4).

Table 3.4 SWOT Analysis of Hot Meals at School

Strengths and opportunities	Weaknesses and threats
• Both parents and school management teams consider hot meals for children to be the most valued option.	• Providing hot meals is exclusionary in nature. Eligibility of pupils is determined by the ability of parents to make contributions (either in cash or in kind).
• Having hot meals involves many stakeholders—parents, pupils, teachers, school management, and school administration—thus strengthening their participation and collaboration.	• Cash payments made in installments make planning difficult, which imposes indirect and unforeseen costs on school management. The ever-rising food prices are an additional challenge for this option.
• Providing hot meals enables an emergence of institutional structures such as the welfare or food committees in schools, which provides a good anchor for health and other welfare needs of schoolchildren.	• Where food is contributed in kind, availability is seasonal, implying that the school may not be able to sustain provision of hot meals throughout the term.
• A uniformity in terms of quality, quantity, and type of food served prevents social differentiation among learners, as summarized by one of the head teachers: "Provision of a hot meal is the ideal option because all children would eat the same meal at the same time, which enhances togetherness at school."	• Having hot meals has fuel requirements (firewood) with a resultant negative impact on the environment. However, providing hot meals could be used as an opportunity to mobilize other line sectors for tree-planting campaigns and for introducing fuel-saving stoves in schools or communities.
• Teachers reported increased school attendance among students participating in this modality, including increased learner concentration, especially during the afternoon sessions.	• A lack of organized cooking and food-serving facilities constrains operations.
• Teachers noted that this method enables the school administration to monitor the movement of teachers and pupils during schools hours and hence eases school management.	• A high degree of teacher involvement may result in time lost from instruction.
• Food purchases by the schools from the community boost household incomes of farmers.	• Providing hot meals calls for organized record management systems.
• Involvement of pupils in food production through school farms increases their knowledge and skills in agriculture.	• It definitely calls for greater hygiene standards than were observed.
	• Food storage facilities were nonexistent in almost all schools visited. Head teachers' offices or bookstores were used for this purpose.
	• Providing hot meals has many direct and indirect costs, including cooking utensils, fuel, cooking stoves, kitchen or cooking areas, labor for cooking, school-level logistics management, and costs of providing water.

Source: World Bank data.

Food Vending and School Canteens

Food vending is a supplementary source of food for pupils who are given money by their parents to buy edible items at school during the midmorning or lunch break. In most schools, food vending operates alongside other food options. Participation depends on a child's ability to pay for what is being sold.

Food vending is undertaken as follows:

- The school administration allocates space. This area can be a small room or canteen in the case of Kampala schools or a small part of the school compound where food vendors operate during break and lunch time, as is the case for most rural schools.
- Vending is done by community members, school parents, or even the pupils themselves. In some instances, pupils were found to be involved in food vending, and head teachers reported that pupils use the proceeds to buy scholastic materials such as books, pens, and pencils.

Pictures of Food Vending in Schools

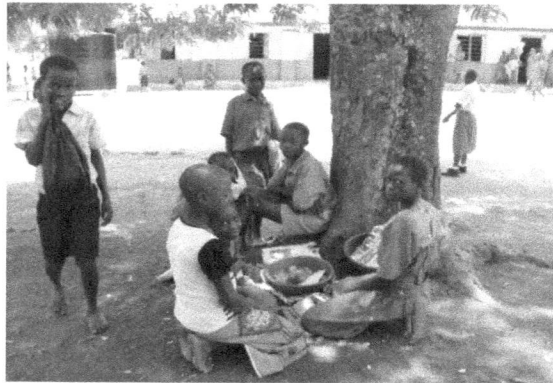

Source: © Mr. Charles Lwanga Bunjo

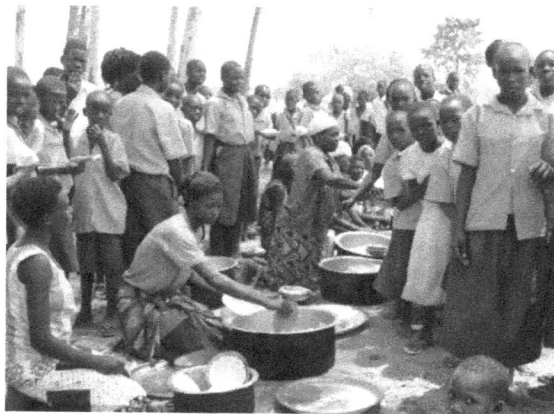

Source: © Mr. Charles Lwanga Bunjo

Pictures of Food Vending in Schools *(continued)*

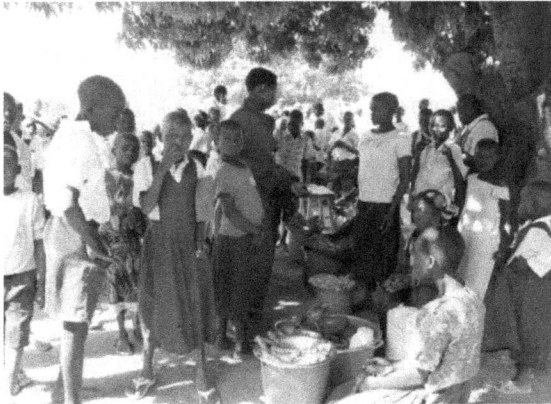

Source: © Mr. Charles Lwanga Bunjo

- Pupils assemble to buy what they find fit for their taste and money. Sellers set prices (ranging from a low of U Sh 300–U Sh 500), and they sell various cooked, roasted, or raw (for example, fruits) food items. The indicated minimum cash requirements imply that children solely using the food vending option would on average spend a minimum of U Sh 72,000–U Sh 120,000 (US$27–US$44) per child per year, if using the standard 240-day school year and assuming that the child takes only one item of not more than U Sh 500 per day.

Type of Food Sold by Vendors

The type of food sold by the vendors depends on the common foods grown in the area and varies by season. The most common items include boiled cassava, beans mixed with maize, banana fingers (*katogo*), ripe banana pancakes (*kabala-gala*), simsim balls, and groundnuts. Fruits, including ripe bananas, jackfruits, mangoes, and sugarcane, were also on sale in a number of schools.

Food Preparation and Serving Arrangements

The following observations were made:

- The respective vendors prepare at home the food they sell at school, and hence the school system cannot ascertain its quality.
- Individual vendors use local transportation modes and incur transport costs to the vending places.
- Vendors carry the food in metallic (saucepans for hot food items) or plastic (for cold food items) containers to the official transaction point at the school.
- Hot food items are served from plates provided by the vendors, and pupils eat the food served at the vending area.
- Food containers were placed mostly on bare ground or grass without any elevated stands or surfaces.
- Most vending places lacked water.

Table 3.5 SWOT Analysis of Food Vending and Canteens at School

Strengths and opportunities	Weaknesses and threats
• Food vending creates a minimal responsibility for the school management team. It is managed outside the school system and hence is less prone to external interference. • It complements other school feeding options, which provides room for schools to address some of the pupils who would be excluded from other in-school arrangements. • It boosts community incomes because the suppliers are from within the community.	• Poor food-handling practices were observed with implications for food quality and hygiene standards. • Schools and parents have difficulty ensuring food quality and standards because they have little or no control over the sources of the vended food. • It is an expensive option for low-income households because it calls for parents to provide daily cash to their children. • It may be exploitative to learners if schools do not help regulate maximum charges for the items sold. • Ensuring the safety of money given to children to buy food is difficult. Often, children steal from each other, or they may lose their money, which calls for security measures at the school level. • When pupils are involved in food vending, it interferes with their concentration in class with a likely negative impact on learning outcomes, notwithstanding the need to meet their educational needs.

Source: World Bank data.

A SWOT analysis reveals the following strengths and weaknesses of the food vending modality (see table 3.5).

Returning Home for Lunch by Pupils

None of the visited schools considered having pupils return home for meals as a school feeding strategy. However, most schools visited had a few pupils go back home for lunch, especially those with homes not very far from schools. The study team could not establish the average distance or time spent between the school and homes. This option works only in schools where pupils are allowed to leave the school compound during lunchtime. The emerging view from the respondents is that whether pupils actually find food when they return home for lunch is difficult to ascertain.

When asked whether going back home for lunch would be feasible, some of the pupils in the focus group discussions indicated the following:

- "By lunchtime, my mother is still in the garden and lunch is not ready," said a pupil of Amolator Primary School.
- "I would spend more time at home because I have to wash the utensils and hence would be late for the afternoon classes," said a pupil of Kotolut Primary School.
- "We have one meal at home in the evening when we are all back, so going back for lunch would not be helpful," said a pupil of Makerere Primary School, Kampala district.

Figure 3.4 Percentage of Primary Pupils Who Go Home for Lunch; QEI Baseline, Uganda 2009

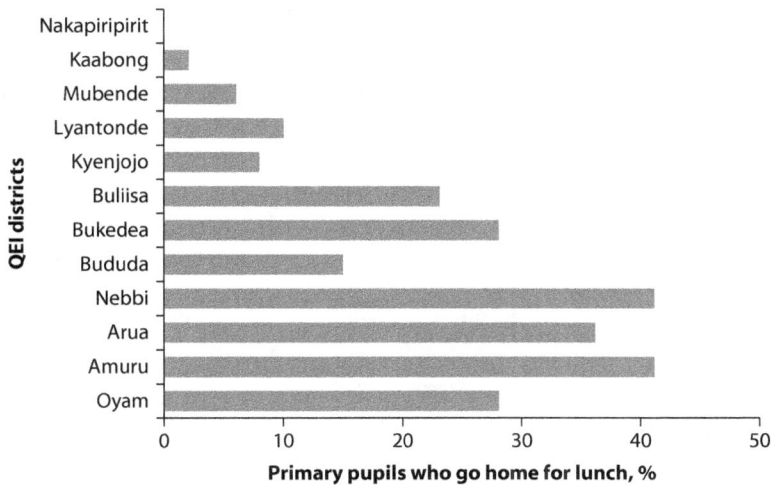

Source: Data from Quality Enhancement Initiative Baseline Survey, Uganda.

Table 3.6 SWOT Analysis of Pupils Going Home for Lunch

Strengths and opportunities	Weaknesses and threats
• Going home for lunch bonds pupils to their homes during school time. • It promotes food security at the household level because parents would have to ensure that food for the children was available by the time they return for lunch. • It is managed at the household level and hence does not create management pressure at the school level. • It is not prone to external influence because it is undertaken in the confines of the household.	• Going home for lunch was reported to be a source of student indiscipline by the head teachers because some pupils leave school to rummage through community gardens instead of going home, which often results in disciplinary cases. • Guaranteeing children's return to school after a home lunch is difficult. This modality could easily contribute to half-day school attendance and to students' subsequently dropping out of school. • The movements to and from school during the school day were cited as a factor that could predispose learners to various sociocultural vulnerabilities, including child sacrifice (for the young ones) and early sexual activity (especially for the upper-primary girls).

Source: World Bank data.

As shown in figure 3.4, the 2009 QEI survey observed that the incidence of returning home for lunch by pupils was highest in Nebbi and Amuru districts (41 percent), followed by Arua district (36 percent). The zero incidences in Nakapiripit and Kaboong districts may be explained by the ongoing WFP program. Of importance is that this option depends greatly on distance traveled by learners to and from school. The UNHS 2009/10 estimated that 73 percent of primary education pupils attended schools within a distance of 3 kilometers, so going home for lunch during the one-hour lunch break may not be feasible for many.

A SWOT analysis of this school feeding option revealed the following strengths and weaknesses (see table 3.6).

Community Contributions to Externally Supported Initiatives

Contributions are not limited to community-led initiatives but are also made to externally supported school feeding programs.

Under the government of Uganda's WFP program, for example, schools in the Karamoja region are supplied with maize flour, corn-soya blend (CSB), beans, sugar, and cooking oil while using the WFP procurement and transportation system. Those supplies enable all supported schools to provide morning porridge of CSB to all pupils between 7 and 8 a.m. of each school day, which is before they begin lessons. Solid food (maize meal and beans) is also provided to all children for lunch and is normally served between 1 and 2 p.m. of each school day.

In addition to hot meals provided at school, girls from P4 to P7 are given take-home rations (THR) as long as they have studied three-quarters of the term. The package includes 25 kilograms of CSB and 5 liters of cooking oil. The THR also serves as a socioprotection strategy for the girls of Karamoja so they complete at least the primary school cycle. The program supplies utensils such as saucepans and plates in addition to food, as well as assistance toward the construction of energy-saving stoves for efficiency and environmental protection purposes.

To complement this package, a cash contribution of U Sh 1,500 per child is made, which supports the food preparation process including firewood purchase and salary payment for the cooks. Most schools under this program were reported to have two cooks, indicating that provision of food to schools is not an end in itself. Other food management processes have to be undertaken at the school level to facilitate meal provision to children at the right time and in sufficient quantities.

A SWOT analysis of this school feeding option revealed the following strengths and weaknesses (see table 3.7).

The study also found that some nongovernmental organizations support school feeding initiatives in selected schools. For example, the Child Health Support Organization supports Kibuuka Memorial Primary School of Mpigi district in school feeding of orphans and other identified vulnerable children by meeting their food requirements at no cost for the children. Other children in the school contribute cash for the semisolid meals. Mission for All supports a school feeding program in Bishop Brown Primary School of Kayunga district. However, these contributions are very isolated initiatives, and few schools have the opportunity of receiving special support from nongovernmental organizations.

The Millennium Village Project (MVP) is an initiative of the United Nations Development Programme that aims at working with communities to ensure that they achieve the Millennium Development Goal targets in a comprehensive manner. Isingiro district is one of the MVP districts, and the project has five core areas: health, agriculture and environment, water and sanitation, education, and infrastructure. Under the education core area, the MVP has supported development of school action plans that embrace school feeding in consultation with and participation of parents and the entire community. (See box 3.5.)

Table 3.7 SWOT Analysis of Community Contributions

Strengths and opportunities	Weaknesses and threats
• Such contributions enabled children in the Karamoja region to realize their right to education, especially girls. • This option contributed to increased levels of access to and quality of education in the Karamoja region. • It is a good model of geographical targeting for the vulnerable, on the basis of which some lessons could be drawn to guide possible program expansion to other areas. • It is flexible in that parental contributions toward food preparation can be made in various ways, including cash, in-kind contributions of firewood, or provision of labor for the direct cooking of the food for the children at school. • The food basket contains well-balanced food for children, and quantities provided are consistent with the daily food requirements of school-age children. • Food quality and preparation norms are standardized, and all children are given one uniform meal in school, which eliminates social differentiation.	• Sustainability of this program by the government is still a challenge.

Source: World Bank data.

Box 3.5

Millennium Village Project in Itungu Mixed Primary School of Isingiro District

One of the schools that has benefited from the Millennium Village Project (MVP) is Itungu Mixed Primary School. This school is located in Nyakitunga subcounty, Isingiro district, in southwestern Uganda.

Through the MVP, the school administration reached an understanding that has enabled the school to provide one midday meal to pupils.

• Parents contribute 5 kilograms of beans per pupil per term.
• Three of the 5 kilograms of beans per child are given to the MVP by the school administration, meaning that the school retains only 2 kilograms of beans per child per term.
• In return, the MVP provides to the school maize flour that is equivalent to the worth of 3 kilograms of beans contributed per child by the school.
• With the beans and maize flour, the school provides a hot midday meal to pupils.
• Pupils who fail to meet the contributions are excluded from the MVP school feeding program.
• The MVP is applauded for the ability to help establish the link between school feeding and the food production chain at the community and family levels.

Although parents contribute beans, they are not part of the process of converting the beans into maize flour for food at school, which was the major identified weakness for this program.

Source: World Bank data.

CHAPTER 4

Emerging Issues for Consideration

This chapter discusses issues that the government needs to consider in attempting to address the school feeding challenge in Uganda.

Coverage of Community-Led Initiatives

The coverage of community-led school feeding initiatives is on average still very low. Table 4.1 shows that except for the schools supported by the World Food Programme (WFP) and some urban schools, all observed options elsewhere had extremely low coverage within the respective schools. A comparison between urban and rural areas reveals relatively better coverage in the urban areas (municipalities and Kampala city division schools) largely because cash contributions toward school feeding are officially instituted, openly discussed, and agreed to by the school management and administrative organs consistent with the agreed modalities of Universal Primary Education (UPE) provision in those settings, which is also articulated in the Education Act of 2008.[1]

The same modality is considered favorable for rural schools by district authorities, school administrations, and parents talked to in the survey. However, the highly politicized nature of school feeding in Uganda has closed the space for open dialogue around this issue at various levels, a factor that has partly contributed to the parental and community failure to execute their role in school feeding. This situation limits the bulk of rural schools mostly to the packing of meals and to food vending options. The low uptake of food packing by pupils (see table 4.1) points to household constraints, ranging from unavailability of surplus food and packaging materials to unsuitability of available food for packing. Similarly, participation in the food vending option depends on parents being able to provide daily cash to children. Schools still have a major challenge of how to effectively engage parents to support school feeding. Parents can fulfill this role only if they are allowed to freely choose what is desirable, affordable, and convenient to them for ownership and sustainability of school-level feeding operations.

Table 4.1 Selected Schools by Region, Enrollment, and Coverage of the Observed School Feeding Option, Uganda 2011

Region and district	Primary school visited	Enrollment 2010/11	Coverage (%)	Location (urban/rural)	Feeding option
South Western Kabale	Kabale Primary School	1,750	287 (16.4)	Urban	Hot meal with solid food, packing from home, going home, or buying from nearby kiosks
	Kitumba Primary School	715	n.a.	Semi-urban	Packing
	Rwere Primary School	495	150 (30.0)	Rural	Hot meal or porridge, packing from home
South Western Isingiro	Ntungu Mixed Primary School	342		Rural-MVP school	Hot meal with solid food for lunch (posho and beans)
Western-Kibale	St. Thereza Primary School	718	n.a.	Urban	Packing (almost all pack)
	Kitutu Parents' School	179	n.a.	Rural	Packing
East-Central	Madibira Primary School	2,014	1,200 (59.6)	Urban	Hot meal of both porridge and solid food for lunch
Busia	Mukwanya Primary School	385	54 (14.0)	Rural	Hot meal with porridge or solid food lunch and porridge for P1 and P2, food vendors
Eastern	Bukedea Primary School	832	50 (6.0)	Urban	Hot meal, food vendors
Bukedea	Kotolut Primary School	700	150 (21.4)	Rural	Hot meal with solid food for lunch
North Eastern Nakapiripirit	Nakapiripirit Primary School	733	733 (100.0)	Urban	Hot meals with porridge for breakfast and solid food for lunch (WFP)
	Napianenya Primary School	406	406 (100.0)	Rural	Hot meals with porridge for breakfast and solid food for lunch (WFP)
Central 1 Kayunga	Bishop Brown Primary School	1,005	337 (33.5)	Urban	Hot meal with porridge and solid food for lunch
	Bulawula Primary School	851		Rural	Hot meal or porridge, food vendors
Central 2 Mpigi	Kibuuka Memorial Primary school	546	200 (36.6)	Peri-urban	Hot meal or porridge and solid food for lunch
	Muduma Catholic School	541	159 (29.4)	Rural/peri-urban	Hot meal or porridge for lunch

(table continues on next page)

Table 4.1 Selected Schools by Region, Enrollment, and Coverage of the Observed School Feeding Option, Uganda 2011 *(continued)*

Region and district	Primary school visited	Enrollment 2010/11	Coverage (%)	Location (urban/rural)	Feeding option
Kampala Kawempe	Makerere Primary school	492	492 (100.0)	Urban	Hot meal with porridge (P1 and P2) and solid food for upper primary
Kampala Rubaga	Kasubi C/U Primary School	1,300	1,300 (100.0)	Urban	Hot meal with porridge (P1 and P2) and solid food for lunch (P3–P7)
Northern Amolatar	Amolatar Primary School	1,287	n.a.	Urban	Food vendors who sell food at break and lunch
	Kataleba Primary School	374	n.a.	Rural	Hot meal or porridge but had not started for the term
West Nile Maracha-Nyadri	Bura Primary School	1,596	35 (2.2)	Peri-urban/rural	Hot meal with solid food (Ugali, which is cassava flour mixed with sorghum, and beans), food vendors, going home at lunch
	Ambekua Primary School	1,361	81 (6.0)	Rural	Hot meal (Ugali), food vendors

Source: World Bank data.

Note: WFP = World Food Programme, n.a. = not applicable.

Flexibility for Responsiveness to Sociocultural and Other Contextual Issues

In light of the various access criteria for the respective community-led options, the survey team observed that most schools that are struggling to ensure food provision to learners depended on more than one feeding method. No fixed pattern of combinations of school feeding options was noted. However, close observation indicated that food packing by learners and hot meals prepared with support from parental contributions (cash or in kind) appeared to be the desirable core options, which are complemented by vended food and outputs of school gardens, where they exist. The multiplicity of approaches tried indicates the need for flexibility in the approaches that schools can use to enable parents and schools to provide children's meals and to respond to household welfare heterogeneity. Smithers (2011) stresses that stakeholder participation has two dimensions: (a) the expression of opinions by citizens and other relevant parties (voice) and (b) the responsiveness of government and other public entities to those opinions. The continued failure, especially by rural schools, to widely adopt the home-packed food option clearly expresses their desire for other options. The government's response by opening up space for other options could thus be a positive step worth considering.

Successful implementation of the community-led feeding program depends not only on the level of community awareness and the value given to education, but also on the sociocultural acceptability of various options in the communities. For example, packing of food, which is perceived to be a generic option, is abhorred in the West Nile region because of sociocultural issues compounded by the fear that children could easily be poisoned by potential family enemies. The survey also found that some staple foods are more easily packed than others. For example, cassava and potato-eating areas find the food-packing option very convenient because those are food items that can easily be eaten cold and without sauce; yet millet, banana, and maize-eating areas find food packing inconceivable because those food items are culturally served hot and require sauce.

Similarly, rural farming communities find the in-kind food contributions convenient compared to nonagricultural or urban settings. This finding, however, does not mean that in-kind food contributions as a modality should be dictated for all rural agricultural areas, because the type of food contributed is another factor that deserves consideration in the successful implementation of this modality. Dry rations such a rice or corn as well as millet and cassava flour were more acceptable and convenient in-kind contributions than were fresh tubers like potatoes and cassava, which not only have short life spans and hence are harder to store, but also are more laborious in preparation (they involve peeling and washing).

Likewise, high-income communities—irrespective of economic activity undertaken—may find cash contributions easier to handle than food packing or in-kind contributions. Again, some pupils indicated that food packing is for the lower- rather than upper-primary grades, which is an aspect that school communities may use in determining what suits them. All these issues are central to the continuity and scaling-up of school-level operations and call for school-level flexibility and autonomy. The center may consider just setting a broad framework on the basis of which sociocultural specifics within districts or even schools can be accommodated. This strategy would form a good base for adaptation and adoption of the Home-Grown School Feeding Initiative in Uganda; with greater potential to increase household incomes as is the case in Ghana and many other countries in the region (see box 4.1).

Smoothly running multiple methods of feeding requires some mechanisms of harmonization and standardization to enable optimal benefits for the children, as well as evolution of management structures for effective and efficient operations. For example, local governments (districts and subcounties) could be given mandates of setting the types of food and standardizing quantities of food to be contributed, or even of setting maximum cash ceilings that could be contributed to schools per child, in consultation with school management teams. Such mandates

Box 4.1

School Feeding Benefits the Local Economy

In Ghana, 80 percent of the feeding costs for children are spent in the local economy through the purchase of locally grown food stuffs for children in school. Registered benefits include increased enrollment, improved school attendance, and significant educational achievement and cognition. The program is also commended not only for the nutritional benefits to the children and community but also for the provision of entrepreneurial opportunities across the supply chain as well as income for small holder farmers.

could help with avoiding wide variations in contributions among schools within the same districts or smaller administrative areas such as subcounties.

Refocus of the Debate on School Feeding

For one to perceive the current low scale of community and parental participation in school feeding as being synonymous with the parents' and community's incapacity to finance the feeding of their children would not be accurate to a substantial degree. The Uganda National Household Survey (UNHS) 2009/10 findings on household assets indicate that 75 percent of households in Uganda possess land. The percentage of households with land was lowest in Kampala (41 percent), and highest was in the eastern and western regions (82 percent and 85 percent, respectively). The proportion of households reporting that food shortages and famines were major problems faced by communities was only 4 percent. Furthermore, 81 percent of the population is rural and earns a living on subsistence agriculture. Those statistics show that the policy position that parents should provide food to learners was justified and has a strong socioeconomic anchor.

Such a low parental response, therefore, deserves more attention. However, the focus has centered more on (a) the mandatory nature of requiring parents to pack food for their children whether or not they would prefer other options than packed meals and (b) the illegal nature of cash payments to schools by parents under the universal education programs, whether or not the management committees to which school management powers were devolved have generated consensus with parents and the wider community. Unlike those in urban schools, the school feeding operations observed in rural schools were reported to be covert in nature, except for packed meals and school gardens, which makes reaching reliable conclusions on the parental capacity aspects impossible.

It is also evident that all school feeding options (both community led or externally supported) have a cost attached to them, as indicated in table 4.2. The only variation is who bears the cost or at what level the cost is borne. This conclusion implies that the debate should shift from paying or not paying for the feeding of

Table 4.2 Cost Elements of Various School Feeding Options

School feeding option	Examples of cost elements	Level at which the cost is realized (not who meets the cost)
Packed meals	Food production or purchase	Household
	Food preparation time	Household
	Food packaging materials	Household
	Food storage space before consumption	School
Hot meals	Food items or cash contributions	Household
	Cooking utensils	School
	Transportation costs for either purchasing items or processing	School
	Labor for cooking	School
	Storage management	School
	Processing	School
	Food serving	School
	Cooking kitchens	School
	Water	School
	Cooking fuel	School

children at school to the realities of *what* should be contributed, *when* (with what regularity), *by whom* (to enable built-in safety nets for the vulnerable, *how* (including management aspects), and *why* (efficiency issues of the various options). The government should thus consider giving the School Management Committees (SMCs) autonomy to generate consensus with parents in partnership with the Parents and Teachers Associations (PTAs). The government needs to support the SMCs' lead in this dialogue by issuing guidelines to provide clarity on possible options, roles of key players, and institutional setups.

Costs of School Feeding

What it takes to implement a national school feeding program also deserves attention so that the government addresses the current state of affairs from an informed stance. Costs of school feeding programs depend on different factors, including choice of modality, composition and quantity of meals, whether the food is locally produced or imported, number of beneficiaries, and number of school days per year. Estimating actual costs is not straightforward, especially for in-school hot meals, because providing them includes a range of school-level costs that could easily be omitted. A recent study by Galloway et al. (2009) estimated the full costs of onsite meal programs (drawing on experience in The Gambia, Kenya, Lesotho, and Malawi) at an average of US$40 per child per year (costs ranged from US$28 to US$63); commodity costs (food items and auxiliary materials) accounted for 59 percent of the total expenditure. The WFP average unit cost for the food program in the Karamoja region of Uganda is estimated at US$50, and this cost includes food, transportation, operational costs, and overheads.

Table 4.3 Estimated Costs of School Feeding by DEOs and Head Teachers of Selected Districts, Uganda 2011

District	Name of primary school	Type of meal	Estimated cost of feeding by DEO/DIS (U Sh)	Estimated cost by head teachers (U Sh)	Average estimated costs/ term (U Sh)
Busia	Madibira	Solid meal	30,000	25,000	27,500
		Porridge	n.a.	15,000	
	Mukwanya	Solid meal	30,000	30,000	30,000
		Porridge	n.a.	15,000	n.a.
Bukedea	Kotolut	Solid meal	10,000	10,000	10,000
	Bukedea	Solid meal	n.a.	30,000	n.a.
Maracha	Ambekua	Solid meal	90,000	60,000	75,000
	Bura	Solid meal	n.a.	50,000	n.a.
Isingiro	Ntungu Mixed	Solid meal	30,000	21,000	25,500
Amolatar	Amolata	Solid meal	60,000	35,000	47,500
	Kataleba	Porridge	n.a.	30,000	n.a.

Source: World Bank data.
Note: DEO = District Education Officer, DIS = District Inspector of Schools, n.a. = not applicable.

In addition, this survey probed some District Education Officers (DEOs) and head teachers about what they consider to be the per term cost of feeding a child in school. Table 4.3 provides a summary of those estimates. The perceived estimates have been averaged; for a solid meal, the range is from a low of U Sh 10,000 per term (U. Sh 30,000 per year) in Bukedea district to a high of U Sh 75,000 per term (U Sh 225,000 per year) in Amolator. The interdistrict diversity in average costs points to the complex nature of standardizing costs because the district-specific estimate probably embraces intrinsic differences in food prices across locales, to which a national estimate may be blind. Within districts, the perceived costs of school feeding reported by the district authorities were higher than those reported by the head teachers, except for Bukedea district. The differential may reflect not only assumed food prices but also perceived management costs that respective parties incur in the entire school feeding exercise either at school for the head teachers or at district level for the district education authorities. Nevertheless, the narrowness of this margin compared to the interdistrict margin reflects the fact that harmonizing costs within schools of the same district is easier than harmonizing across districts.

Table 4.4 provides insights about the likely costs of school feeding on the basis of various unit costs per pupil in Uganda. The estimates are not in themselves conclusive. Rather they are meant not only to direct decision makers about the indicative cost margins but also to bring to the fore issues of cost implications of such an undertaking at only the primary level for an informed way forward.

The feasibility of the government meeting any of the costs in light of the current financial constraints faced by the education sector—largely arising from

Table 4.4 Estimated Costs of School Feeding on the Basis of Various Indicative Unit Costs (in US$) per Pupil in Uganda

Years	Target group (all children ages 6–12 in primary[a])	Unit cost of food at $40[b] discounted at 5%	Net discounted total annual costs	Unit cost at lowest estimate of DEOs of $12.60[c] discounted at 5%	Net discounted total annual costs	Unit cost of US$9.60[d] estimate of MoES for a semisolid meal discounted at 5%	Net discounted total annual costs	WFP unit cost of US$50 discounted at 5%	Net discounted total annual costs
1	6,037,601	$38.10	$230,003,847.62	$12.00	$72,451,212.00	$9.14	$55,200,923.43	$47.62	$287,504,809.52
2	6,236,842	$36.28	$226,279,975.80	$11.43	$71,278,192.38	$8.71	$54,307,194.19	$45.35	$282,849,969.75
3	6,442,658	$34.55	$222,616,395.24	$10.88	$70,124,164.50	$8.29	$53,427,934.86	$43.19	$278,270,494.05
4	6,442,658	$32.91	$212,015,614.51	$10.37	$66,784,918.57	$7.90	$50,883,747.48	$41.14	$273,765,162.24
5	6,442,658	$31.34	$201,919,632.87	$9.87	$63,604,684.35	$7.52	$48,460,711.89	$39.18	$269,332,773.90

Source: World Bank data.

Note: DEOs = District Education Officers, MoES = Ministry of Education and Sports, WFP = World Food Programme.

a. Enrollment statistics of the first year are based on the 2009/10 Uganda National Household Survey (UNHS) weighted estimates of children ages 6–12 in Uganda, and this cost has been projected to increase by 3.3 percent, consistent with the population growth rate for Uganda.

b. The average annual cost of onsite school feeding per child per year of US$40 was estimated by Galloway et al. as reported by Bundy et al. (2009) and was based on experience in The Gambia, Kenya, Lesotho, and Malawi. The estimate provides insights on what actual costs would be for a national program.

c. Lowest estimate of DEOs and head teachers of U Sh 10,000 per term = US$4.20 per term = US$12.60 per year.

d. Lowest estimate of U Sh 100 = US$0.04 per day for a semisolid meal of a cup of porridge as provided in the draft Cabinet Memo on school feeding.

the implementation of the ongoing primary and secondary universal education reforms—is low. For example, if one uses the least-cost proposal by the education sector of providing only one cup of porridge to pupils per day, then that daily estimate of U Sh 100 (US$0.04) translates into U Sh 24,000 (US$9.60) per child per year. This cost implies that at least US$55 million would be required to implement a national program in the first year. Although this estimate is 80 percent lower than the regional average estimate of US$40 per day per child, it is 3.5 times higher than the primary pupil's annual capitation grants provided to schools.

Increasing the budget levels of the capitation grants to such a magnitude may thus not be feasible. Should the government opt for funding levels that are close to what is considered moderate by the district officials and head teachers, at least US$72 million would be required for a national program in the first year, while cost estimates close to the regional unit cost average or WFP costs in Uganda would call for at least US$259 million. In addition, sustainability challenges of externally led initiatives have been reported everywhere; hence, the opportunity of leveraging families and communities could be taken advantage of by the government consistent with the provisions of the Education Act as indicated in chapter 2. Government support may be extended to only the most vulnerable, as discussed in the next chapter.

Responding to Social Shocks and Targeting the Excluded

School feeding is not only an educational but also a social protection strategy. The social safety net roles of school feeding initiatives include an immediate response to social shocks, as well as social protection over a long period of time (Bundy et al. 2009). Geographical targeting is the most frequent explicit criterion used in centrally led school feeding programs on the basis of food insecurity as well as the educational context (identification of areas with the greatest educational need). Profiling is often at subnational units such as districts or regions. A case in point here is that the WFP in Karamoja is not only targeting a geographically poor and educationally underserved region but also addressing the social vulnerability of girls through the take-home rations (THR) component of the program within the same region.

The observed community-led school feeding options all depend on the status of households and hence have an inherent element of exclusion because households are prone to many socioeconomic shocks. Results from the 2009/10 UNHS data indicate that 24 percent of the children ages 6–12 had stopped attending school because of a calamity in the family including sickness and death (see figure 4.1). Double orphanhood is a widespread phenomenon among school-age children in Uganda and is largely caused by parental AIDS deaths. In addition, the disruption of households from natural calamities (mudslides or floods) has become the norm in some parts of the eastern region, all of which suggest that learners from affected families

**Figure 4.1 Percentage of Pupils Ages 6–12 Who Left School Due to Calamity in Family,
UNHS 2009/10**

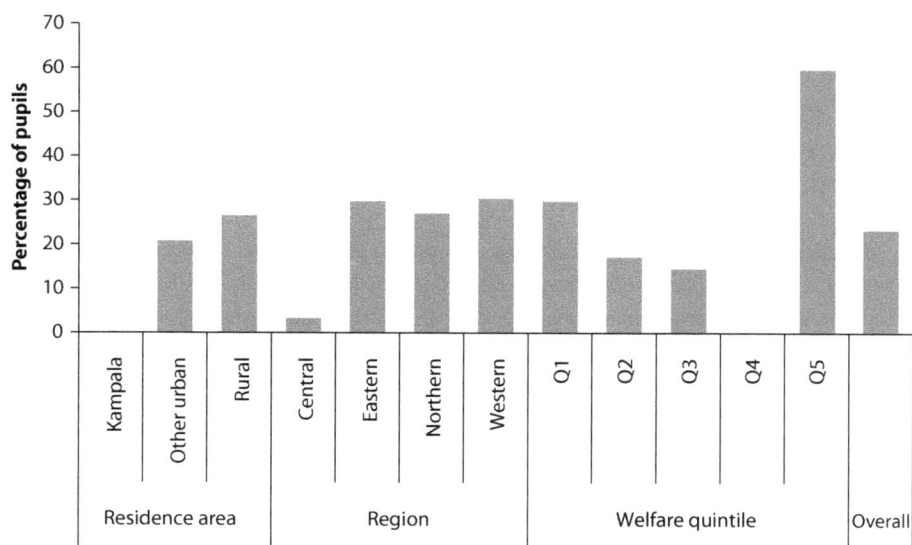

Source: Data from the Uganda Bureau of Statistics.

would need to be protected from short-term hunger while at school.
Children from extremely poor households also may not be able to meet their
school feeding requirements through the community-led approach and
hence cannot take advantage of the available free education services for a
better future. Therefore, the key question is this: how can schools support
affected learners in adjusting to normal family eating patterns without dis-
rupting learning?

Schools have no provisions for addressing learners from households that
may be affected by various socioeconomic shocks within the current framework. Individual school-level targeting would be the most useful for the
school systems in this regard. It is context dependent, and identification is
done within the community setting while relying on inputs from multiple
stakeholders. If the government considers providing some resources to schools
for individual excluded children, then proxy means testing (PMT) would need
to be developed. PMT should draw from the village and school levels because
local institutions tend to be more accountable to the people, thus weaving
into school systems and subnational levels thereafter through to the national
level for effective planning and budgeting. Good practices in this regard can
be drawn from Bangladesh (Galasso and Ravallion 2005) and Chile (Kain,
Uauy, and Taibo 2002), and their success has been attributed to the long-term
nature through which those programs have been evolving since the 1960s (see
Box 4.2).

Box 4.2

Resources in Chile, Bangladesh, and Malawi

In Chile, primary schools are provided free school meal allocations on the basis of a school vulnerability index that relies on socioeconomic household data of first-grade schoolchildren. The index determines the cutoff (also guided by the available fiscal budget) and the amount of food received by the school. Importantly, in Chile, the food provided is considered "a benefit that allows vulnerable children to have equal opportunities in the education system," and it is not in any way intended to be universal. A committee decides who receives the meal on the basis of the school-level learners' data. Teachers are then asked to target free meal allocations to the most vulnerable in the classrooms while all other children get the meals at a cost. Coverage was estimated at 40 percent by 2001, and the program was targeting about 2.2 million children per day by 2009.

In Bangladesh, a similar targeted school feeding program is being undertaken. In January 2011, an additional targeted school feeding program was launched for urban working children ages 10–14 in Dhaka.

The Malawi government plans to support primary school-going children in vulnerable schools through what is called the Targeted Support to School Meals Program.

Source: World Bank data.

Table 4.5 shows potential beneficiaries of social protection through school feeding in Uganda according to the UNHS 2009/10 data. If one were to go by the 24.5 percent poverty rate, close to 29 percent of the primary school population could be considered eligible for support. The proportion is, however, much higher for the rural areas (30 percent) than in the urban areas (20 percent) and the Kampala district (7 percent). Other finer criteria could be used by identifying the poor within the most vulnerable subgroups for more affirmative action. Here are examples: poor double orphans (28 percent); poor children with disabilities (about 30 percent); and poor children displaced because of insecurity (57 percent), drought (50 percent), and land evictions (30 percent).

Figure 4.2 shows consumption dominance curves of the second order for potential beneficiaries and draws on the respective selection criteria presented in table 4.5. The curves are useful in assessing the effect of a subsidy on poverty, as demonstrated by Makdissi and Wodon (2002) and Duclos, Makdissi, and Wodon (2008). When using consumption dominance curves of the second order, one is, in practice, considering the effect of subsidies on poverty measures such as the poverty gap. Such consideration takes into account not only the share of the poor in the population, but also the distance separating the poor from the poverty line, or the "depth" of poverty (when computing the poverty gap, the nonpoor are included in the estimate, but they are given a zero distance separating them from the poverty line because they are not below that line).

Table 4.5 Potential Beneficiaries of Social Protection through School Feeding in Uganda, UNHS 2009/10

	Total	The poor using the 24.5% poverty rate	% of poor	The poor using the 40% poverty rate	% of poor
Population (ages 6–12)	7,236,333	2,066,061	28.6	3,266,596	45.1
Kampala	248,557	16,297	6.6	34,633	13.9
Urban	594,043	118,684	20.0	190,978	32.1
Rural	6,393,734	1,931,081	30.2	3,040,985	47.6
Potentia. beneficiaries of social protection (individuals)					
Children ages 6–12	7,236,333	2,066,061	28.6	3,266,596	45.1
Children ages 6–12 in primary	6,037,601	1,621,857	26.9	2,633,883	43.6
Girls ages 6–12	3,592,346	991,081	27.6	1,591,440	44.3
Girls ages 6–12 in primary	3,032,776	792,297	26.1	1,306,443	43.1
Children ages 6–12 living without their father	798,020	274,078	34.3	381,741	47.8
Children ages 6–12 living without their mother	366,501	109,822	30.0	159,129	43.4
Children ages 6–12 living without both parents	188,557	52,173	27.7	80,732	42.8
Disabled 1 (strong)	57,202	18,868	33.0	25,027	43.8
Disabled 2 (soft)	172,417	53,714	31.2	75,193	43.6
Displaced by land eviction	2,606	788	30.2	1,317	50.5
Displaced by drought	1,666	837	50.3	1,047	62.8
Displaced by insecurity	141,566	80,265	56.7	98,242	69.4
Children ages 6–12 who ate no breakfast yesterday	1,609,081	603,706	37.5	889,086	55.3

Source: Data from the Uganda Bureau of Statistics.

The effect of the subsidy on poverty reduction among identified popula-tions is established by ordering the dominance curves for the respective groups. If one consumption dominance curve is above another, then the subsidy's effect on poverty reduction of that particular subgroup is high, and the subsidy provided for it deserves to be increased while reducing a subsidy for the population that corresponds to the curve that is located below it in that order.

On the basis of the data on potential beneficiaries, where the curves repre-sent dummy variables, the consumption dominance curves of order two actually represent the share of beneficiaries who are poor. The horizontal axis represents the level of consumption per equivalent adult normalized by the poverty line, so that a value of one corresponds to the poverty line that is actually used in Uganda. In figure 4.2 for example, at a value of one on the horizontal axis (which means that one is looking at the share of beneficiaries that are poor), the value of the horizontal axis for the displaced due to insecurity is about 56 percent. This means that the poor as a whole, who are 28.6 percent of the population ages 6–12, constitute about 56 percent of those children displaced due to insecurity.

Figure 4.2 Cumulative Dominance Curve for Potential Beneficiaries of School Feeding, Order 2, Uganda 2009/10

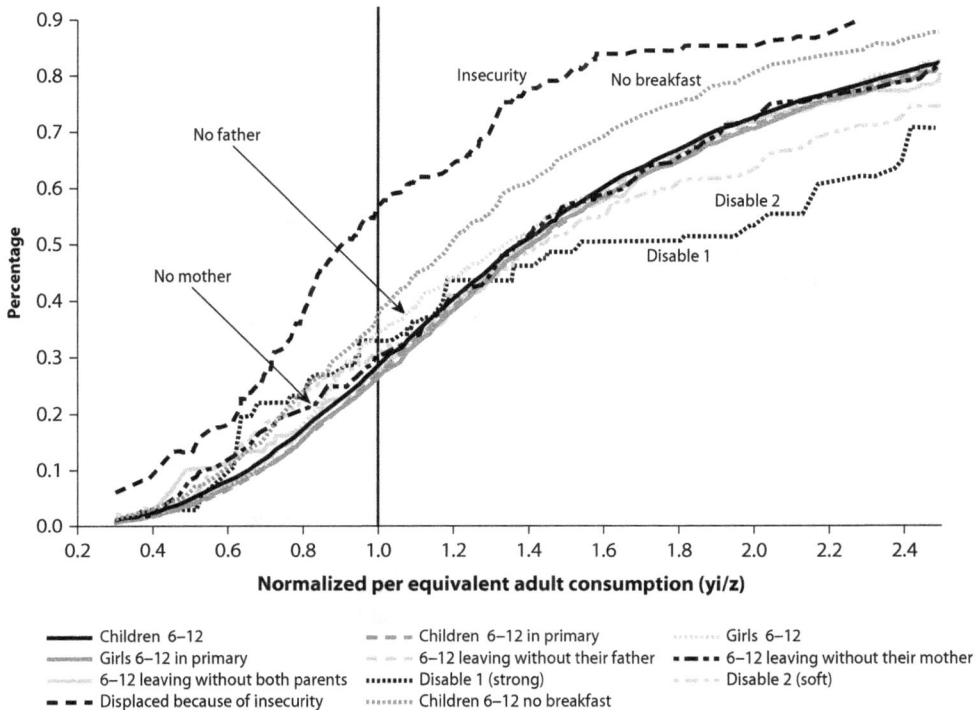

Source: Data from the Uganda Bureau of Statistics.
Note: yi = household welfare indicator, z = poverty line.

In terms of comparing the various potential beneficiaries and curves in figure 4.2, girls who are ages 6–12 in primary school and children ages 6–12 in primary school have the lowest curves. This observation means that the poverty rates among girls ages 6–12 in primary school and among children ages 6–12 in primary school are lower for any poverty line to the left of 1.4. Above 1.4 of the official poverty line, the groups with disabilities have the lowest curves. In contrast, groups displaced because of insecurity, those who had no breakfast, and orphans have the highest curves. Thus, if a subsidy toward school feeding or poverty reduction among children ages 6–12 were feasible for Uganda, school-going children displaced because insecurity, those who no breakfast, and orphans would be best to target, because this targeting would have a higher effect on the poor and on poverty. Appendix B provides annual cost estimates for the respective target groups to provide insights to the government and to potential development partners and stakeholders in this undertaking.

Further analysis on how such groups could be more accurately identified was undertaken while using the 2009/10 UNHS data. Modalities used could be either geographic (regional or district) or PMT. An estimate was made of errors of inclusion (identifying nonpoor persons as poor and therefore admitting them to the program) and errors of exclusion (identifying poor persons as not poor and thus denying them access to the program) for both modalities. The relevance of the district as a geographical area in this analysis arises from the decentralized nature of education service delivery in Uganda, and the statistics would be more appropriate for district-level planning.

Because of the greater seriousness placed on errors of inclusion under limited-budget situations, as is the case for Uganda (related to share of benefits going to the poor), the analysis of errors conducted indicates that the best way of identifying those to be targeted would involve using a combination of PMT and geographical criteria within districts regardless of the level of capital expenditure below or slightly above the poverty line (see figures 4.3–4.6, and the tables in appendix A).

After one identifies potential target groups, exploring the various means of reaching them with subsidies for school feeding is important. These means would greatly depend on objectives of the intervention, economics of food consumption among the poor, capacity requirements relating to the administrative needs of various modalities, efficiency and cost-effectiveness, and beneficiary preferences for enhanced ownership. An attempt is made next to highlight two modalities that the government may consider: direct disbursement to schools

Figure 4.3 Estimates of the Errors of Inclusion at 11 Percent of the Target Populations, UNHS 2009/10

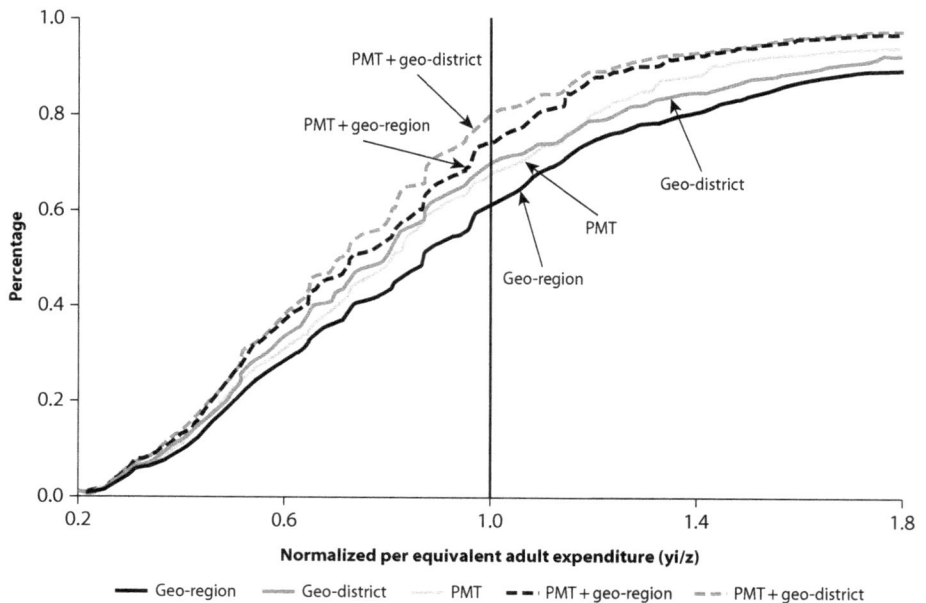

Source: Data from the Uganda Bureau of Statistics.
Note: yi = household welfare indicator, z = poverty line.

Figure 4.4 Estimates of the Errors of Inclusion at 22 Percent of the Target Populations, UNHS 2009/10

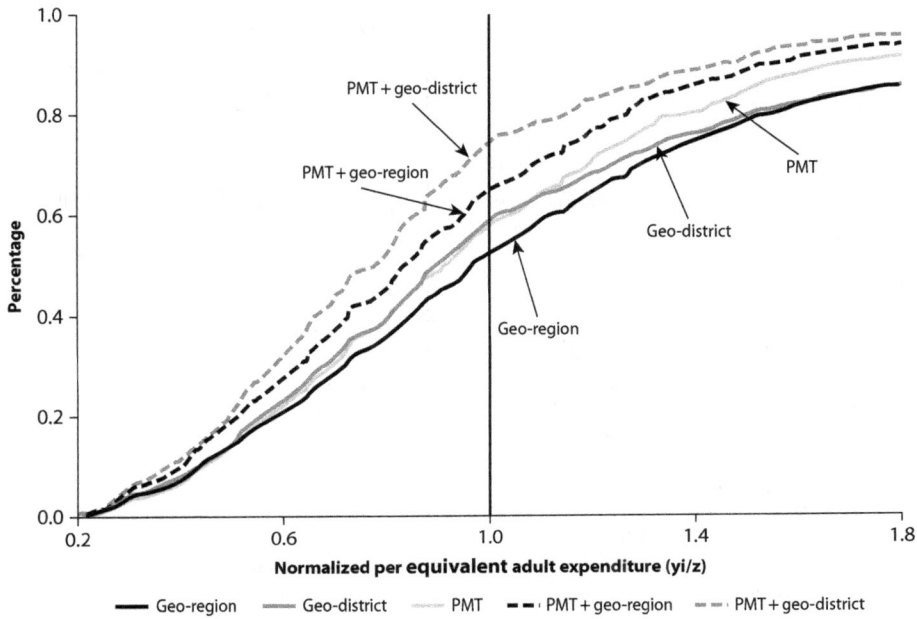

Source: Data from the Uganda Bureau of Statistics.
Note: yi = household welfare indicator, z = poverty line.

Figure 4.5 Estimates of the Errors of Inclusion at 33 Percent of the Target Populations, UNHS 2009/10

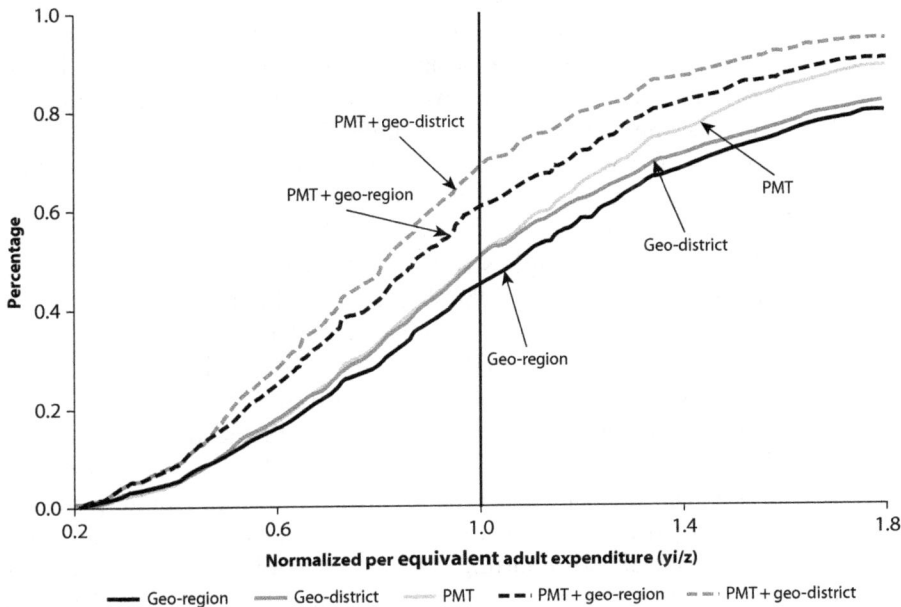

Source: Data from the Uganda Bureau of Statistics.
Note: yi = household welfare indicator, z = poverty line.

Figure 4.6 Estimates of the Errors of Inclusion at 55 Percent of the Target Populations, UNHS 2009/10

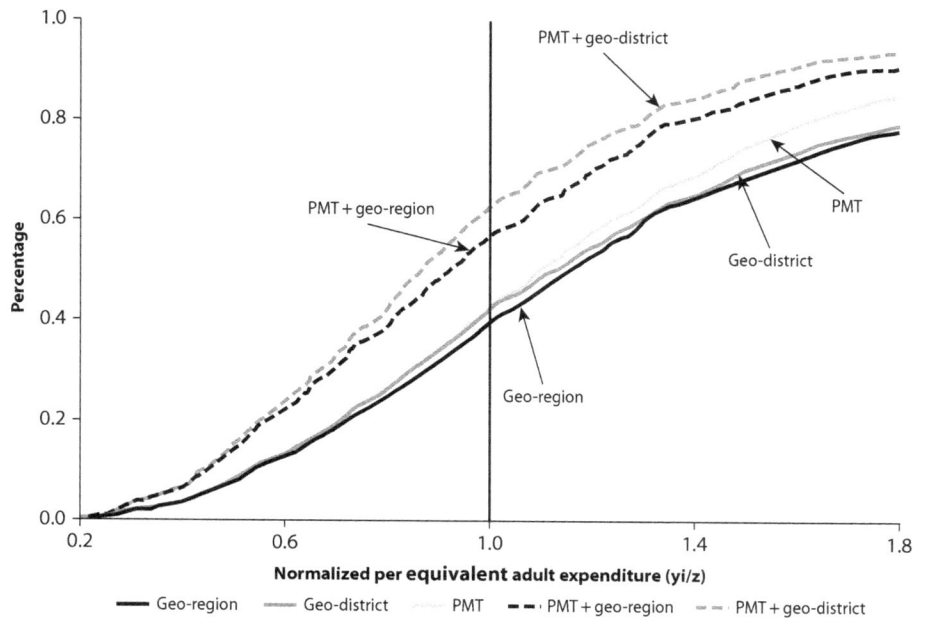

Source: Data from the Uganda Bureau of Statistics.
Note: yi = household welfare indicator, z = poverty line.

and cash transfers. Because this chapter is trying to make a case for targeting the excluded children in schools outside the food-insecure region of Karamoja, which is provided for by the WFP/government of Uganda (GoU) initiative, food aid or in-kind food transfers may not be appropriate and are not discussed here.

Direct Disbursement to Schools. The government disburses capitation grants to schools to facilitate the implementation of UPE. The grant constitutes a minimum threshold amount that is allocated to each school according to the standard nature of some costs regardless of school characteristics. In addition, the schools receive an annual enrollment-based allocation that is an aggregate of the learner-specific grant and currently stands at U Sh 7,000 per child (US$2.50). The government's contribution to school feeding of the most vulnerable children may thus be provided to schools through a similar mechanism; the school feeding grant could be an addition to the funds already provided to schools. This method would require establishing an acceptable sum per child, which would be based on which budget allocations would be made and on how disbursements to schools were effected. The use of existing disbursement mechanisms has advantages, which include (a) no requirement to develop system processes and financing, and (b) outright integration of the financing mechanism in the already existing financial and reporting systems and guidelines. What would be missing is the guidance to schools about the targeting mechanisms or identifiers of the most vulnerable, with higher chances that those identifiers could vary depending on household welfare dynamics. The involvement of the SMCs in this process could also be easier to mobilize.

Cash Transfers. The use of cash transfers to targeted poor or food-insecure households with school-age children is another funding arrangement that the government could explore. Cash transfer programs have been regarded as an effective way to reconcile safety nets with investments in human development that would benefit the poor and, hence, would be of high relevance to the agenda for improving learning in Uganda under universal education programs. Cash transfers are justified by the assumption that individuals can be trusted and empowered to make effective use of resources available to them to improve their living standards (Arnold and Conway 2011). In addition, cash is considered to be economically more efficient (Tabor 2002) and provides recipients with freedom of choice and a higher level of satisfaction at any given level of income than in the case of food or any other type of in-kind transfer (Subbarao et al. 1997).

Cash transfers have been regarded as a leading-edge social policy tool because of their ability to influence both income and human capabilities of the poor, including making easier the integration of different types of social services, such as health and education (Kakwani, Soares, and Son 2005). Whether the transfers should be conditional or unconditional is a design issue and hence not discussed at this stage. Modest but regular and reliable flows of income from cash transfers help households smooth their consumption. Available evidence indicates that cash transfers in African countries that have been studied significantly contribute to reducing hunger and food insecurity, as well as improving school enrollments and attendance. Severely impoverished households that receive additional income are particularly likely to prioritize their spending on the basis of improving the quantity or quality of food consumed. Cash transfers can also be an important complement to direct education investments. Increased income security enables households to pay fees or other costs associated with attending school (see also box 4.3).

A number of challenges with implementation of cash transfer programs have been identified, which should guide the government's decision making. Not all transfers given to households are spent on children. The real value to the beneficiaries may erode with inflation, yet the government's nominal budget is always fixed and predictable. It is thus important that the real budget keeps pace with inflation (Akhter, Quisumbing, and Hoddinott 2007). The high administrative costs of cash transfer programs is another common criticism, because a substantial volume of resources is spent on getting the resources to the poor families (Kakwani, Soares, and Son 2005), compounded by the need to obtain the necessary accurate estimates of household income or consumption. Gelb and Majerowicz (2011) indicate that Uganda is far from being able to implement the policy of transfers to individuals in light of existing systemic issues, including weak local capacity and accountability challenges.

Box 4.3

Cash Transfer Programs in Brazil and Mexico

Brazil's *Bolsa Escola* conditional cash transfer program started in 1995 and was aimed at increasing school attendance and curbing dropouts. Today, under the coordination of the education ministry, monthly payments are made to poor households with children ages 6–15 and enrolled in grades 1–8 on the condition that they had at least 85 percent school attendance. The size of transfers is between US$5 and US$15 per household. Overall estimates are determined nationally using an agreed poverty line per month per household. Implementation is left to local levels with some variations. In some places, beneficiaries are selected by schools, while other areas use geographical criteria. Administration of the transfers was contracted to a commercial bank.

Mexico's *Progresa* started in 1997. It is a comprehensive program for education, health, and nutrition and is aimed at alleviating poverty and promoting human development. It consists of cash and in-kind transfers to beneficiary households. Those transfers to households are conditional on school attendance of children up to the age of 18 and on regular visits to health centers by all the household members. By 2003, the size of the transfer ranged from US$10 to US$60, depending on the program component and the beneficiary children's grade and gender. Administration of transfers is managed through various channels, including organizations and banks.

Source: World Bank data.

Nevertheless, one pilot model could serve as a guide to what needs to be done if the government adopts this financing modality. The Action against Hunger Food Security and Livelihood Intervention is one example. It was implemented in Otuke district in 2009 and used unconditional cash transfers targeted at the 1,500 most vulnerable households in 34 villages, facilitated by the district's Equity Bank Branch. Training of beneficiaries was also undertaken. An external evaluation in mid-2010 indicated that the project's effect on the livelihood assets for households was significant. Eighty-four percent of the grant had been spent on productive assets—particularly livestock—and 16 percent on immediate needs. About 54 percent of the funds for immediate needs went to food. The effect of the program on the local economy was also seen as significant. The study concluded that at least half the funds passed directly to farmers with medium-size holdings in Otuke. Those farmers were the main sources of the livestock purchased as well as ox-plows and other income-generating items (see Pietzsch 2011). Worth noting is that the private sector plays a key role in implementing effective cash transfer programs.

Although targeting individual children on the basis of need can produce considerable benefits in cost-effectiveness, especially where central or external intervention is planned, Bundy et al. (2009) highlight potential social costs from stigmatization and hence the need for strong buy-in from the community to minimize the negative effects of individual targeting.

Reliance on School Gardens for School Feeding

School gardens are often used in conjunction with other school feeding arrangements and may thus not be sufficient to provide food requirements for learners year-round. Also important is that adoption of food production through school gardens depends on availability and size of school farmland and water. In addition, two boxes (3.3 and 3.4) presented in this report signal the need for high-level commitment on the part of school management and communities.

Where higher yields were observed in the WFP-supported school, intensive support (for example, inputs or food items for participating parents) was provided to schools and parents. Consistent with this observation, Foeken, Owuor, and Mwangi (2007) found that school gardens in Kenya were more successful in schools that already had school feeding programs and reported more inputs (both local and improved seeds, pesticides and fertilizers, irrigation), some of which were externally provided. All this observation implies that school gardens are not cost-free. Realization of substantial outputs depends greatly on the inputs and commitment, the inadequacy of food provision notwithstanding.

School gardens, therefore, are not sufficient to sustain school feeding programs, and caution is needed to ensure they do not detract from the teaching and learning goals for which they are established. School gardens are broadly meant to provide experience to children on sustainable agricultural production coupled with the use of improved and locally appropriate technology and nutrition prospects. Products often include diversified food crops, fruits, vegetables, and weather-resistant varieties of grain and staples that may be used to complement the food provided under different schemes within schools. (Guidance by the FAO on how to establish School gardens exists as shown in box 4.4).

Box 4.4

Additional School Gardening

The Food and Agricultural Organization (FAO) of the United Nations has put in place information materials on how to set up school gardens for use in schools (for example, "Setting Up and Running a School Garden: A Manual for Teachers, Parents, and Communities"). Wider dissemination by FAO of this type of information to schools could be useful.

The ongoing initiative titled "A Thousand Gardens in Africa," with 14 participating schools in Mukono and Kayunga districts where the Terra Madre network operates, could model good practices. Lead teachers could be engaged in sharing experiences with other schools for wider adoption, especially the concept of sustainable farming models.

Source: World Bank data.

Food Quality and Hygiene Standards

The quality of food provided in school feeding programs was noted to be low. In all food arrangements observed, most food is bulky starch of low fat and protein content with low nutritional value in terms of protein content and calories, and meals were not balanced. None of the feeding options deliberately provided vegetables, fruits, and animal protein on the children's menu despite the small numbers served. Common foods are maize, cassava, potatoes, beans, and sorghum (for the West Nile region). Carbohydrates are filling and have high satiety value, and beans are good sources of vegetable protein and iron. However, vegetable proteins are normally considered incomplete proteins because they do not have all the essential amino acids. In many cases, pupils' meals often miss some important nutrients such as vitamins and minerals such as calcium. The most common methods of food preparation are boiling and steaming. Only in the WFP-supported program was cooking oil provided. Fruits were almost nonexistent in the observed schools.

Table 4.6 provides information about the daily recommended dietary intake for primary school pupils. Developing a school-based program that meets all those requirements would not be easy. However, Galloway (2010) states that providing at least one-third of the daily energy requirement is a viable goal in many developing countries. Specific to Uganda, the WFP already has computations of the nutrient composition per 100 grams of edible portions of local and commonly eaten foods, which is a good starting point for schools.

Food hygiene standards were observed to be very low regardless of the school feeding option. Schools had inadequate infrastructural provisions for food storage and preparation. In addition, pupils rarely practiced hand washing, which was constrained in some settings by unavailability of water. Soap was not found in any of the schools visited. Food utensils were often improvised, and

Table 4.6 Recommended Daily per Capita Dietary Intake for Primary School Pupils

Dietary content	Age category		
	Preprimary 3–5 years	Primary 6–12 years	Adolescent 11–14 years
	1. Energy and Safe Protein Intake		
Energy (Kcal)	1,700	1,900	2,350
Protein (grams)	32	40	46
	2. Vitamins and minerals		
Vitamin A (ugretinol/IU)	400/1,330	400/1,330 to 500/1,665	600/2,000
Iron (mg)	10	10	12 (boys)
			15 (girls)
Iodine (mg)	90	120	150

Source: Adapted from UNESCO FRESH Tools for Effective School Health 2004 (http://www.unesco.org/education/fresh).

Box 4.5

Health Training in Ghana

In Ghana, a series of trainings are organized for school cooks and caterers by the Ghana Health Services at various levels, with an aim of imparting knowledge and skills that enhance kitchen safety and hygiene, food hygiene, and storage standards. The training also provides information about nutritionally balanced meals.

Such training events provide opportunities for the target group to undergo medical checkups. This activity enables identification and, where possible, treatment of communicable diseases, thereby reducing the risk of their transmission to children.

Source: World Bank data.

their care was generally inadequate. General environmental sanitation, including human excreta disposal facilities, was inadequate in most visited schools. This situation calls for training in food quality and hygiene for those involved in food preparation and for the community at large (see box 4.5).

Complementary and Multisectoral Approaches

Feeding children in school can improve participation; alleviate short-term hunger; and increase children's ability to concentrate, learn, and perform specific tasks. Evidence suggests that integration of complementary interventions such as deworming and micronutrient supplementation has potential to augment educational benefits, because good health and nutrition are prerequisites for effective learning. Strengthening mechanisms for control and prevention of micronutrient deficiencies through promotion of supplementation (vitamin A, iron, and zinc), deworming, and food fortification with essential micronutrients is one of the identified strategic objectives of the National Development Plan within the health theme.

Infection with common roundworms and bilharzias (schistosomiasis) tends to be most prevalent and intense in school-age children (Bundy 2005). Therefore, regular deworming contributes to good health and nutrition of school-going children, which in turn leads to increased enrollment and attendance. Programmatic evidence indicates that deworming through schools is safe, cheap, and remarkably cost-effective. In a randomized controlled trial in Kenya, deworming was found to increase school participation by 7 percent, amounting to a 25 percent decline in total absence (Miguel and Kremer 2004). Promising new research suggests that deworming children can result in many long-term benefits, including higher wages, healthier individuals, and stronger communities (Bundy 2011).

Box 4.6

Multisectoral Programs

Common implementation steps of multisectoral school-based health programs include (a) determining whether a school is at risk on the basis of epidemiological information available; (b) determining a strategy for mass treatment in keeping with the World Health Organization's recommendations; (c) training teachers and providing information to the community; (d) procuring drugs and materials; (e) treating targeted in school children; and (f) monitoring and evaluating the programs, including routinely recording basic information such as the number and percentage of children treated and the drug quantities as required by the public health system.

Ghana's complementary activities to school feeding include school-based deworming and nutrition education, which provides opportunities to address health problems of schoolchildren in a comprehensive manner.

Zambia's program of feeding urban poor students is complemented by an human immunodeficiency virus (HIV) and acquired immune deficiency syndrome (AIDS) component and by school-based agriculture through which students grow nutritional foods like vegetables, fruits, and poultry production is promoted.

Source: World Bank data.

To the extent possible, the food should be fortified with minerals and vitamins to generate benefits on the nutritional and learning outcomes front. As earlier mentioned, all the feeding arrangements observed provide mostly bulky starch of low fat and protein content, with the exception of the WFP-supported program. Vegetables, fruits, and animal protein were also not provided, which could be a cost issue compounded by insufficient knowledge about food value and a lack of open dialogue around school feeding issues in schools.

Food fortification at the point of use just before consumption is an emerging technology where hot meals are prepared at school. Micronutrient powder has been used in food-based programs in emergency situations and is currently being piloted in Tanzania and Cambodia, as well as other countries (Hamdani 2008). In Uganda, the Micronutrient Strategies and Technology program, which supports food fortification for private education providers, could be extended to public schools to support community-led initiatives.

For improved learning outcomes, the government, through the Ministry of Health in partnership with the education sector, may consider designing and implementing a school health program package including all the elements previously highlighted to supplement parental contributions (see box 4.6). Multisectoral programs like this would greatly enhance the operationalization of the Focusing Resources for Effective School Health (FRESH) partnership framework and would further the collaboration among various stakeholders, including (a) development agencies that are working on education and health, (b) education and health managers and practitioners at various levels in the field, and (c) parents and school management teams, as has been the case elsewhere. Various cost sources indicate that school-based health interventions fetch an average annual per capita cost of about US$0.50 (for example, between US$0.03 and US$0.20 for deworming drugs, US$0.04 for vitamin A supplementation, and US$0.30–US$0.40 for iodine supplementation), with anticipated high economic returns through improved health outcomes and high productivity. The rise in productivity is through higher levels of cognitive ability that enhance school participation and years of schooling attained. The draft School Health Policy for Uganda embeds this framework. It should thus be passed and resourced for implementation to actualize these elements in schools.

Operational Arrangements, Including Roles and Responsibilities

Evidence from chapter 3 signals that school-level operational arrangements deserve attention. The multiplicity of players involved in implementing community-led school feeding activities, together with their regular and intensive engagement in this undertaking, offsets the stress at various levels and grounds the sustainability bid. Local factors such as eating habits; availability of food in the community and at household level; ease of food preparation; shelf life of local food items; availability of personnel to support the school-level activities related to food provision (food preparation, serving, cleaning up); costs (for example, fuel and wages for cooks); and availability of safe water sources, cooking facilities, and eating or packing facilities all feature in the various school feeding options. The need to coordinate is imperative for efficient running of community-led school feeding programs, as seen from the roles of the respective players as highlighted in table 4.7.

The few schools visited indicated the existence of school-level institutional structures either in the form of committees (food management committees or welfare committees) or through a focal point person, normally the deputy head or the teacher in charge of welfare. The composition of committees varies, but membership commonly observed includes the welfare teacher, representatives from the SMC, parent representatives, and student leaders. As is the case with other school-level committees, the representation and roles of these committees need to be streamlined and harmonized to allow full evolution of community-led school feeding schemes. The importance of the committee is mostly to serve as the interlocutor between the parents and community, on the one hand, and the school management and administration, on the other hand, in the overall management of the school feeding schemes. In addition, the committee ensures efficient use of food or resources pertinent to the food program. Areas of concern include the need for the

Table 4.7 Roles and Responsibilities of Various Players

Parents	Pupils	School management and administrative team	Local government leadership
• Provide materials (for example, food, money, utensils, firewood, and food packaging materials). • Mobilize and encourage fellow parents to participate in a community-led feeding scheme. • Participate in the management of feeding schemes, including planning, monitoring, and supervising.	• Play generally minimal roles, often at the point of food preparation and serving, except where they engage in food vending activities for purposes of improving welfare. • Contribute labor in preparing and serving of food (for example, by bringing firewood, sorting maize, serving, and fetching water). • Play supervisory roles, especially prefects at mealtimes in some schools. • Disseminate information to parents or guardians in case of emerging changes at school in regard to respective school feeding options.	• Initiate and plan the feeding arrangements. • Sensitize and mobilize parents to participate in the arrangement. • Perform everyday management of the scheme (school administration), which may vary depending on the nature of the feeding options. • Provide liaison with district officials and development partners (in case of externally supported arrangements).	• Provide direction about school feeding at the district or lower-level unit consistent with the Education Act, UPE policy, and local government norms (bylaws, ordinances, or resolutions). • Mobilize communities to take up various modalities. • Monitor compliance. • Articulate emerging issues at council or other high level for action.

Source: World Bank data.

Note: UPE = Universal Primary Education.

committee to ensure that teachers do not take over the overall management of the feeding program because that action has serious opportunity costs. For example, where teachers are responsible for food preparation, serving, or even purchasing of food and other related items, it is likely to affect their time on task and thus reduce learning. Excluding teacher participation should also be seen as a protective measure in situations of potential mismanagement of the scheme. In Mali, for example, management of school feeding programs was devolved to PTAs (see box 4.7).

Box 4.7

Responsibilities in Mali

In Mali, the management of school feeding supplies is undertaken by the PTA, including maintenance of cooking facilities. The strategy has been successful, especially in regard to community ownership. The PTA, in turn, provides regular reports on the program to the school management team.

Source: World Bank data.

Planning for Sustainability

With the low coverage of the ongoing initiatives partly explained by lack of clarity from the government, considering the future of school feeding in Uganda is important. Most of the school feeding literature about future planning focuses on possible exit strategies from externally supported programs. The most common option for countries is establishing national school feeding programs that are mainstreamed into the national policy including transition from externally supported to national projects, as has been the case with WFP-supported programs in more than 28 countries. Although the case of community-led initiatives is different to some extent, their transition to long-term sustainable schemes including supportive mechanisms and institutional frameworks still needs to be projected.

Community ownership and mainstreaming of initiatives into national plans and structures are some of the principles of sustainability. The existence of community-led school feeding initiatives reflects the ownership bid by the school community, including the inherent demand, its thin operational scope notwithstanding. Clarity on what are considered to be approved or appropriate modalities would greatly benefit household- and school-level planning and implementation of those initiatives. Uganda's decision to devolve this role to parents and communities places it at a higher scale on the sustainability continuum. The only challenge that remains is to ensure nurturing of the partnership with communities and parents to reinforce the already built-in sustainability bid.

The widely reported politicization of feeding children in school was identified as a contributor to the lack of clear district and school-level plans on school feeding. This situation is compounded by the lack of guidelines, which weakens reinforcement by the school administration. All options need to be planned for by either parents or school management for effective operations and sustainability. A number of issues deserve consideration, some of which are highlighted next.

- The sustainability of community-led initiatives hinges on the continuous availability of food at the household level (a) to pack for the child, (b) to provide to the school in kind (corn, millet, and beans), or (c) to sell to children through a vendor. Planning for household food security thus emerges as being central to the sustainability of school feeding programs and for creating links between education and agriculture. Such plans are a good entry point for the adaptation and adoption of the home-grown school feeding framework within the Uganda community-led school feeding model.
- Cash contributions require planning not only at the household level, where income sources have to be identified, but also at the school level. Planning for cash contributions will enable an accurate projection of needs vis-à-vis charges to be levied per child, all of which will be based on operational and future food prices and costs of auxiliary elements. Observations indicate that costs are not accurately estimated at this time. Because of the prevalent fear about the illegal nature of charging pupils for food, the amounts set are more symbolic than

realistic, which partly explains the insufficiency of contributions and the resultant on-and-off patterns of these schemes.

- Clarity on acceptable modalities could inform community mobilization plans and development of school-level structures, which would be one way of ensuring sustainability of the various initiatives. It would also trigger open dialogue and lesson learning across schools and communities, elements that are currently missing from these initiatives.
- Providing social safety nets to children who are currently excluded from school feeding programs, as discussed earlier, calls for planning if effective and efficient implementation of supplemental school feeding programs is to be undertaken.

All in all, these initiatives can be sustained only if clarity exists on what they should be to enable their effective integration into national, household, and school-level plans. Only then will clear cost elements, actors, and responsibility centers be identified and resources allocated at appropriate levels through satisfactory and consultative means. The current situation does not allow the evolution of such processes to sustainable levels despite the inherent potential embedded in the demand from communities and parents and the favorable legal framework that devolves this role to parents and communities.

Accountability and Procurement Monitoring

Procurement mechanisms are central to the success of the community-led school feeding options if additional modalities other than home-packed meals are to be given a chance to thrive. Systematic tendering and bidding processes are used most frequently in large procurements outside or within the country. For lower administrative levels such as schools with small but regular transactions involving school feeding, bidding may not be appropriate or even possible, but this situation does not mean that food operations are not susceptible to abuse if badly managed. Therefore, a need exists for a transparent process with broad community involvement to safeguard communities from abuse that could generate negative perceptions about the viability of feeding schemes. Local food procurement systems have the potential to develop community food production and processing capacity. They would also enable variations in the school food basket according to seasonal food availability and would provide schools the potential for price negotiations and optimal use of their resources. Transportation and logistics as well as storage capacity may pose constraints in some areas, however.

Learning from school experiences with community-supported infrastructure development programs, which have always been applauded, the government can mandate school-based structures to develop simple, flexible, transparent, and satisfactory procurement modalities for feeding programs. The structures should clearly separate potential interest groups with a desire to benefit from preferential markets or even potential political influence. Inflows and outflows from the food budgets have to be regularly reported. In large urban schools, a combination of different procurement modalities may be used that weave into nationally approved modalities according to the items being procured. For example, an urban school may want to upgrade to electric cooking pots, which are not produced in Uganda, if it considers such pots more efficient than the local alternatives currently used.

Environmental Concerns

Even though the operations are still small in scale, their potential expansion has a bearing on the environment. The preparation of in-school meals requires the use of fuel and will involve the use of wood and charcoal from the adjacent areas, thereby contributing to deforestation over time. Between 1990 and 2005, Uganda's forest cover outside protected areas was reduced by 1.2 million hectares (from 3.46 to 2.3 million hectares), and the annual deforestation rate is estimated at 1.8 percent (NFA 2009). In addition, the value of the charcoal and firewood consumption at household level increased more than tenfold between 2005/06 and 2009/10 (UBOS 2011). The two aspects call for household and school-level planning in this area. Learning from the ongoing WFP/GoU-supported projects, schools can promote fuel-efficient cooking stoves (through dissemination of different designs that are based on local technologies), and tree-planting around schools can be promoted elsewhere with the involvement of communities and school management.

The planting of woodlots with WFP/GoU support in schools is worth replicating elsewhere through links with the environmental management and forestry subsectors. The effort can also be extended to the household level. For example, learners can be urged to plant at least 5 trees a year, implying at least 35 trees planted per child by the end of the primary education cycle. This is one of the areas where private sector involvement through socio-cooperative responsibility or even politicians' constituency funds could be leveraged by schools or households. Such a program would yield long-term environmental gains while supporting the fuel needs of school feeding initiatives. In some countries (for example, Belize [Raimer 2002][), tree planting is an integral part of school gardening. Reusable food sacks can also be encouraged for use in schools. Multisectoral links may allow leveraging of tree seedlings and construction of fuel-efficient stoves for some schools. Availability of standard designs for the latter is of great importance.

School-Level Infrastructure

Shortage of supportive school-level infrastructure was noted in all schools. The lack of permanent kitchens or cooking space, storage facilities, and utilities such as water compromises food quality and hygiene standards. Low-cost designs for this infrastructure need to be developed by the Construction Management Unit to guide school management teams in resource mobilization drives such as have been used for community-supported infrastructure development in schools. Their existence is as important as other school infrastructure for quality learning environments.

Monitoring and Evaluation

Community-led school feeding initiatives need to be integrated in the mainstream monitoring and evaluation system of the Ministry of Education and Sports (MoES) along with other line sectors that would be undertaking activities complementary to school feeding in schools. Clear and measurable indicators that capture different modalities by target group for respective schools need to be developed. A system of monitoring and evaluation is a key aspect for ensuring sustainability of these operations. To develop this aspect, MoES could use the existing school feeding monitoring and evaluation toolkit that was developed under the thematic subgroup of Focus Resources on Effective School Health (FRESH) partners.

Political Will

Political will is central to the promotion and scaling-up of community-led school feeding initiatives in Uganda. Some of the core indicators of political will in this case would be (a) government efforts to initiate or actively support community-led school feeding schemes, (b) response to attempts to articulate underlying constraints to the one school feeding model (food packing) for rural schools, (c) creation of open dialogue platforms at school level to explore and implement other mechanisms for improving parental performance of their school feeding roles, and (d) enforcing sanctions for nonperformance. Using these elements, the current rating for Uganda's political will to promote community-based school feeding schemes would be considered low. Political leadership at all levels should commit itself to supporting and nurturing the existence of various school feeding schemes in schools for improved learning in Uganda as reflected in their messages and actions. Technocrats also need to ensure that all regulatory instruments and other elements are in place to guide and ensure quality implementation of community-led school feeding schemes.

Note

1. Section 13(1) of the Education Act of 2008 clearly states that no person or agency shall levy any charge under UPE institutions while section 13(2) indicates that the provisions in 13(1) should not be construed to deter school management from collecting or receiving voluntary contributions or payments from parents and wellwishers to contain a state of emergency or any urgent matter concerning the school. The urban schools rely on section 13(2), and parents pay levied charges voluntarily. The last sentence is one of the many instances in the report where it is not clear why rural schools cannot rely on the same subsection.

CHAPTER 5

Conclusion and Next Steps

In conclusion, for improved learning in Uganda, the school feeding challenge could be addressed through the following three actions by government.

Action 1*: Removing all barriers to parental participation in school feeding.*

This could be done through effective promotion of community-led school feeding options to enable schools have a menu of school feeding options for flexibility and sensitivity to regional and household heterogeneity. Political will at all levels, would be required to support these initiatives, together with clear operational guidelines for the various school feeding options including roles and responsibilities of key stakeholders.

Community-led school feeding options have inherent potential to expand into nationally recognized and sustainable school feeding schemes, as well as to increase parental capacity to fulfill this obligation for improved learning in Uganda. Flexibility will remove barriers to establishing modalities for increased parental participation that would be based on what would be desirable for them, thereby resulting in increased coverage and lessening the proportion of children going without lunch during the school day. The immediate result would be anticipated improvements in learner attendance and concentration. Likely added benefits include evolution of strong institutional structures at the school level, more parental ownership, involvement and sustainability of school operations, and increased community incomes because community farmers and markets would service the schools.

Feeding all children by government through a well-coordinated and sustainably resourced national school feeding program is not feasible. The lowest possible funding option of US$9.6 would require an increase in the education sector annual budget of at least 8 percent (see Table 5.1). Other factors such as cost-benefit ratios of school feeding vis-à-vis other school inputs such as teachers and instructional materials, together with other unfunded priorities that are required for effective implementation of the ongoing mass education reforms in Uganda would also need to be accurately projected but that type of analysis is outside the scope of this report. This would also imply that school-level support

Table 5.1 Estimated Costs for a National School Feeding Program in Uganda Excluding Administration Costs in US$

	Unit cost of US$40 per child per annum[a]	Unit cost of US$12.60 per child per annum[b]	Unit cost of US$9.60 per child per annum[c]
Average annual expenditure[d]	218,567,093.21	68,848,634.36	52,456,102.37
% of education budget for FY11/12	33.9	10.7	8.1

Source: World Bank data.

Note: The analysis is based on the enrollment statistics derived from the 2009/10 Uganda National Household Survey (UNHS) weighted estimates of children ages 6–12 in Uganda and is projected to increase by 3.3 percent per year.

a. Unit cost of US$40 is the average annual cost of onsite school feeding per child per year, an estimate based on the experience of The Gambia, Kenya, Lesotho and Malawi (Bundy et al. 2009). The WFP cost for Uganda is US$50 per child per year including administrative costs.

b. Unit cost of US$12.60 is based on the lowest estimate of DEOs and head teachers provided in the survey.

c. Lowest estimate of a semisolid meal (cup of porridge with sugar) is proposed in the MoES's draft Cabinet Memo.

d. Average annual expenditure is based on the computations of 5 percent discounted annual costs over a 5-year period.

infrastructure such as cooking shades and food stores would also be provided by the government. Removing barriers to parental participation would therefore, be the best option for government for an effective and sustainable partnership with parents in the delivery of education.

Action 2: *Targeting those children who are excluded as a result of extreme poverty, food insecurity, and household shocks.*

The observed community-led school feeding options all depend on the status of households and hence have an inherent element of exclusion because households are prone to many socioeconomic shocks. Family calamities like deaths and sickness of parents and guardians; the orphan hood phenomenon largely caused by acquired immune deficiency syndrome (AIDS) deaths; disruption of households from natural calamities; and extreme household poverty; all point to the need for government to attend to the affected children to enable their realization of the right to education. This would hence enhance the safety net role of school feeding. In this regard, various modalities of targeting the excluded could be adopted based on guidance provided in this report.

Action 3. *Designing and implementing a school health program package aimed at provision of complementary school based health programs such as deworming, and food fortification, reinforced by community and parental training on nutritional values of various foods.*

Integration of complementary interventions such as deworming and micronutrient supplementation has potential to augment educational benefits, because good health and nutrition are prerequisites for effective learning. The government, through the Ministry of Health in partnership with the education sector, may consider designing and implementing a school health program package including all the elements previously highlighted to supplement parental contributions. Multisectoral programs like this would greatly enhance the operationalization of the Focusing Resources for Effective School Health (FRESH) partnership framework and would further the collaboration among various stakeholders, including: (a) development agencies that are working on education and health; (b) education and health managers and practitioners at various levels in the field; and (c) parents and school management teams.

Recommendations for Next Steps

Adoption of the above mentioned actions calls for the following immediate steps by the education sector.

1. Initiate dialogue with government to obtain political buy in on the above mentioned actions. Dialogue points include: (a) providing school management teams with powers to dialogue with parents on the various school feeding options available; (b) government's agreement and modalities for catering for the excluded few as a social safety net; and (c) committing resources to support complementary school health programs including implementation modalities.
2. Finalize the draft school feeding guidelines with more clarity on the various school feeding options available to schools for consideration by parents. guidelines will: (a) facilitate explicit and transparent dialogue with parents and various stakeholders; (b) enable evolution of school-specific modalities with clear roles and responsibilities of various players; (c) minimize political interference and give schools more autonomy over their operations; (d) enable development of school implementation plans for the respective school feeding options deemed appropriate and acceptable to the school community; (e) enable accurate monitoring of coverage of various options in the respective areas and provide clarity on constraints that may require local or central government interventions; (f) guide standards setting, including those for food hygiene and quality; (g) guide schools' assessment of their needs where external support could be mobilized, which could also be the entry points for private sector players; and (h) enable initiation of a dialogue about the need to reach out to the excluded children as a social protection strategy, together with development of implementation mechanisms for such a program. This approach would enable harmonized alignment of external support and development partner engagement in such a program beyond the operational scope of the World Food Programme/government of Uganda (WFP/GoU) program in Uganda.
3. Distribute and disseminate the guidelines for wider reach and immediate adoption.
4. Form an interministerial committee on school feeding to address the multisectoral nature of this issue, and enable the design and implementation of

complementary initiatives as well as school feeding programs for the children likely to be excluded. For example, initiatives should include school health aspects (food fortification, vitamin supplementation, and other nutrition issues that are drawn from the draft National School Health and Nutrition Policies); environmental concerns (tree planting and energy-saving stoves); promotion of household food security (agricultural development initiatives); and income generation. Expediting passage of the draft School Health Policy would greatly enhance this process.

APPENDIX A

Table A.1 Errors of Inclusion and Exclusion at 11 Percent

	Error of inclusion					Error of exclusion				
	Geographic-region	Geographic-district	PMT	PMT and geo-region	PMT and geo-district	Geographic-region	Geographic-district	PMT	PMT and geo-region	PMT and geo-district
Children ages 6–12	39.1	30.0	32.1	25.6	20.1	76.5	73.8	66.2	78.3	74.9
Children ages 6–12 in primary	44.7	34.4	34.8	29.6	21.9	80.4	77.2	70.0	82.3	78.4
Girls ages 6–12	41.9	32.4	33.6	28.1	22.4	74.9	72.2	64.6	76.6	73.1
Girls ages 6–12 in primary	45.8	35.6	35.2	30.4	23.6	78.5	75.5	69.2	80.4	76.4
Ages 6–12 living without their father	42.3	34.4	24.2	24.5	24.0	77.6	70.4	64.3	79.0	72.3
Ages 6–12 living without their mother	40.3	36.8	22.7	26.3	24.5	75.5	68.5	56.7	77.8	69.6
Ages 6–12 living without both parents	35.0	37.4	20.4	14.0	23.1	81.0	63.6	49.9	81.0	64.7
Disabled 1 (strong)	58.8	44.2	43.8	65.8	44.2	93.7	93.6	73.7	95.3	93.6
Disabled 2 (soft)	38.4	42.4	32.4	26.7	34.6	89.1	86.3	65.7	91.3	86.3
Displaced because of land eviction	100.0	0.0	0.0	0.0	0.0	100.0	100.0	100.0	100.0	100.0
Displaced because of drought	20.0	20.0	20.0	20.0	20.0	0.0	0.0	0.0	0.0	0.0
Displaced because of insecurity	56.5	31.1	32.0	0.0	22.1	99.2	62.8	49.6	99.2	62.9
Children ages 6–12 with no breakfast	25.3	14.1	33.2	17.3	10.8	79.2	70.8	68.1	80.0	71.7

Source: World Bank data.

Note: PMT = proxy means testing.

Table A.2 Errors of Inclusion and Exclusion at 22 Percent

	Error of inclusion					Error of exclusion				
	Geographic-region	Geographic-district	PMT	PMT and geo-region	PMT and geo-district	Geographic-region	Geographic-district	PMT	PMT and geo-region	PMT and geo-district
Children ages 6–12	47.6	41.0	42.1	35.0	25.5	59.5	56.1	44.3	63.2	62.3
Children ages 6–12 in primary	51.5	43.8	44.4	38.1	26.4	62.5	58.7	47.1	66.3	65.4
Girls ages 6–12	49.8	42.5	44.0	36.7	27.2	58.5	55.2	44.4	61.9	61.2
Girls ages 6–12 in primary	53.2	44.6	46.2	39.2	28.1	61.5	58.1	47.4	65.1	64.5
Ages 6–12 living without their father	47.0	36.9	39.1	33.8	26.0	52.6	49.4	46.5	55.6	58.6
Ages 6–12 living without their mother	50.7	45.5	39.0	37.5	33.5	42.6	45.6	42.1	46.6	51.1
Ages 6–12 living without both parents	48.9	45.5	41.7	33.5	32.0	31.9	40.1	37.2	34.2	42.3
Disabled 1 (strong)	49.9	32.5	32.1	47.5	30.2	78.4	73.4	37.1	80.0	75.1
Disabled 2 (soft)	44.7	38.8	33.3	33.3	26.7	64.9	60.5	44.1	67.1	67.1
Displaced because of land eviction	100.0	100.0	0.0	0.0	0.0	100.0	100.0	0.0	100.0	100.0
Displaced because of drought	49.7	49.7	20.0	20.0	20.0	0.0	0.0	0.0	0.0	0.0
Displaced because of insecurity	41.0	33.5	37.8	35.6	25.7	9.1	23.1	29.3	18.0	29.3
Children ages 6–12 no breakfast	38.3	28.1	42.4	27.0	18.2	57.5	53.1	43.1	60.4	57.6

Source: World Bank data.

Note: PMT = proxy means testing.

Table A.3 Errors of Inclusion and Exclusion at 33 Percent

	Error of inclusion					Error of exclusion				
	Geographic-region	Geographic-district	PMT	PMT and geo-region	PMT and geo-district	Geographic-region	Geographic-district	PMT	PMT and geo-region	PMT and geo-district
Children ages 6–12	54.9	49.3	49.3	39.1	30.8	48.0	41.3	27.8	57.2	52.9
Children ages 6–12 in primary	57.9	51.3	51.3	41.4	31.8	51.1	42.8	29.7	60.5	55.4
Girls ages 6–12	56.1	51.7	50.3	41.2	33.2	47.4	41.1	26.7	56.4	51.3
Girls ages 6–12 in primary	58.3	53.2	52.2	42.6	33.9	49.8	42.9	29.0	59.2	54.1
Ages 6–12 living without their father	46.6	37.4	41.5	35.6	26.3	40.2	34.6	31.7	50.3	49.4
Ages 6–12 living without their mother	53.2	44.1	46.0	41.5	31.6	37.4	32.3	20.2	44.5	39.9
Ages 6–12 living without both parents	51.1	42.0	43.6	38.8	29.3	27.5	19.5	11.7	34.2	21.8
Disabled 1 (strong)	55.5	25.2	26.8	38.4	30.2	65.6	62.1	7.7	70.9	75.1
Disabled 2 (soft)	52.6	44.4	36.6	36.3	27.1	45.3	48.2	17.9	58.0	63.5
Displaced because of land eviction	40.2	100.0	40.2	0.0	0.0	0.0	100.0	0.0	0.0	100.0
Displaced because of drought	49.7	49.7	20.0	20.0	20.0	0.0	0.0	0.0	0.0	0.0
Displaced because of insecurity	41.0	37.2	36.5	35.6	31.7	9.1	2.5	8.4	18.0	14.7
Children ages 6–12 no breakfast	44.1	38.5	45.7	29.3	23.8	48.6	34.5	23.0	54.3	46.3

Source: World Bank data.

Note: PMT = proxy means testing.

Table A.4 Errors of Inclusion and Exclusion at 55 Percent

	Error of inclusion					Error of exclusion				
	Geographic-region	Geographic-district	PMT	PMT and geo-region	PMT and geo-district	Geographic-region	Geographic-district	PMT	PMT and geo-region	PMT and geo-district
Children ages 6–12	60.5	57.9	57.5	43.1	37.0	30.7	25.4	12.6	46.5	43.0
Children ages 6–12 in primary	62.8	60.2	59.4	45.3	39.0	31.8	26.6	13.6	48.5	45.4
Girls ages 6–12	62.1	59.7	59.7	44.9	38.8	30.4	25.9	13.5	44.6	41.7
Girls ages 6–12 in primary	64.0	61.7	61.6	46.8	40.8	31.4	27.3	15.0	46.5	44.5
Ages 6–12 living without their father	49.2	47.2	50.1	35.2	33.4	26.2	21.6	15.4	41.4	41.3
Ages 6–12 living without their mother	53.4	52.7	52.7	39.3	33.0	23.3	20.1	9.4	36.1	32.0
Ages 6–12 living without both parents	52.3	49.9	51.5	36.7	31.6	14.3	5.0	7.9	21.0	15.9
Disabled 1 (strong)	53.5	60.4	44.1	38.4	26.1	57.9	56.5	0.0	70.9	69.5
Disabled 2 (soft)	57.2	59.6	52.3	37.1	33.8	39.0	34.3	0.9	55.3	52.0
Displaced because of land eviction	40.2	40.2	40.2	0.0	0.0	0.0	0.0	0.0	0.0	0.0
Displaced because of drought	49.7	49.7	20.0	20.0	20.0	0.0	0.0	0.0	0.0	0.0
Displaced because of insecurity	41.5	39.8	39.4	35.8	33.6	0.0	0.0	3.4	12.3	12.3
Children ages 6–12 no breakfast	51.9	50.4	51.8	39.1	34.3	24.6	20.9	8.9	39.3	36.7

Source: World Bank data.

Note: PMT = proxy means testing.

APPENDIX B

Table B.1 Estimated Costs of School Feeding for All Children in Primary and Various Target Groups of Children Likely to Be Excluded from Participating in Community-Led School Feeding Schemes (see column 4 of respective tables)

Years	Unit cost of food at US$40	Net discounted unit cost (US$)	Target group (all ages 6–12 in primary school)	Net discounted total costs per year ($)
1	40	38.10	6,037,601	230,003,847.62
2	40	36.28	6,236,842	226,279,975.80
3	40	34.55	6,442,658	222,616,395.24
4	40	32.91	6,442,658	212,015,614.51
5	40	31.34	6,442,658	201,919,632.87

Years	Unit cost of food at US$9.60 estimate of MoES for a semisolid meal	Net discounted unit cost ($)	Target group (all ages 6–12 in primary)	Net discounted total costs per year ($)
1	9.6	9.14	6,037,601	55,200,923.43
2	9.6	8.71	6,236,842	54,307,194.19
3	9.6	8.29	6,442,658	53,427,934.86
4	9.6	7.90	6,442,658	50,883,747.48
5	9.6	7.52	6,442,658	48,460,711.89

Years	Unit cost of food at lowest estimate of US$12.60 estimate by DEOs and head teachers per year	Net discounted unit cost ($)	Target group (all ages 6–12 in primary)	Net discounted total costs per year ($)
1	12.6	12.00	6,037,601	72,451,212.00
2	12.6	11.43	6,236,842	71,278,192.38
3	12.6	10.88	6,442,658	70,124,164.50
4	12.6	10.37	6,442,658	66,784,918.57
5	12.6	9.87	6,442,658	63,604,684.35

Years	Unit cost of food at US$40	Net discounted unit cost ($)	Target group (all poor ages 6–12 in primary)	Net discounted total costs per year ($)
1	40	38.10	2,066,061	78,707,085.71
2	40	36.28	2,134,241	77,432,780.52
3	40	34.55	2,204,671	76,179,106.93
4	40	32.91	2,204,671	72,551,530.41
5	40	31.34	2,204,671	69,096,695.63

Years	Unit cost of food at US$40	Net discounted unit cost ($)	Target group (all poor single and double orphans ages 6–12 in primary)	Net discounted total costs per year ($)
1	40	38.10	436,073	16,612,304.76
2	40	36.28	450,463	16,343,343.64
3	40	34.55	465,329	16,078,737.12
4	40	32.91	465,329	15,313,082.97
5	40	31.34	465,329	14,583,888.55

Years	Unit cost of food at US$40	Net discounted unit cost ($)	Target group (all poor children with disabilities ages 6–12 in primary)	Net discounted total costs per year ($)
1	40	38.10	72,582	2,765,028.57
2	40	36.28	74,977	2,720,261.44
3	40	34.55	77,451	2,676,219.11
4	40	32.91	77,451	2,548,780.11
5	40	31.34	77,451	2,427,409.63

Years	Unit cost of food at US$40	Net discounted unit cost ($)	Target group (all poor girls ages 6–12 in primary)	Net discounted total costs per year ($)
1	40	38.10	792,297	30,182,742.86
2	40	36.28	818,443	29,694,069.88
3	40	34.55	845,451	29,213,308.75
4	40	32.91	845,451	27,822,198.81
5	40	31.34	845,451	26,497,332.20

Years	Unit cost of food at US$40	Net discounted unit cost ($)	Target group (all poor ages 6–12 displaced due to drought, insecurity and land evictions)	Net discounted total costs per year ($)
1	40	38.10	81,890	3,119,619.05
2	40	36.28	84,592	3,069,110.93
3	40	34.55	87,384	3,019,420.56
4	40	32.91	87,384	2,875,638.63
5	40	31.34	87,384	2,738,703.46

Years	Unit cost of food at US$40	Net discounted unit cost ($)	Target group (all poor ages 6–12 without breakfast yesterday)	Net discounted total costs per year ($)
1	40	38.10	603,706	22,998,323.81
2	40	36.28	623,628	22,625,970.00
3	40	34.55	644,208	22,259,644.77
4	40	32.91	644,208	21,199,661.68
5	40	31.34	644,208	20,190,153.98

Years	Unit cost of food at US$40	Net discounted unit cost ($)	Target group (all poor ages 6–12 rural)	Net discounted total costs per year ($)
1	40	38.10	1,931,081	73,564,990.48
2	40	36.28	1,994,807	72,373,938.25
3	40	34.55	2,060,635	71,202,169.73
4	40	32.91	2,060,635	67,811,590.21
5	40	31.34	2,060,635	64,582,466.87

Years	Unit cost of food at US$40	Net discounted unit cost ($)	Target group (all poor ages 6–12 urban)	Net discounted total costs per year ($)
1	40	38.10	118,684	4,521,295.24
2	40	36.28	122,601	4,448,093.32
3	40	34.55	126,646	4,376,076.57
4	40	32.91	126,646	4,167,691.97
5	40	31.34	126,646	3,969,230.45

Source: World Bank data.
Note: DEOs = District Education Officer.

REFERENCES

Adelman, S., H. Alderman, D. O. Gilligan, and K. Lehrer. 2008. "The Impact of Alternative Food for Education Programs on Learning Achievement and Cognitive Development in Northern Uganda." International Food Policy Research Institute, Washington, DC. http://users.ox.ac.uk/~econ0274/downloads/Alderman_Gilligan_Lehrer_FFE__School_Participation.pdf.

Afridi, F. 2010. "The Impact of School Meals on School Participation: Evidence from Rural India." Discussion Paper 10-02, India Statistical Institute, Delhi.

Ahmed, A. U. 2004. *Impact of Feeding Children in School: Evidence from Bangladesh.* Washington, DC: International Food Policy Research Institute.

Akhter, U. A., A. R. Quisumbing, and J. F. Hoddinott. 2007. *Relative Efficacy of Food and Cash Transfers in Improving Food Security and Livelihoods of the Ultra-Poor in Bangladesh.* Submitted to the World Food Programme, Dhaka, Bangladesh, by the International Food Policy Research Institute, Washington, DC.

Alderman, H., D. O. Gilligan, and K. Lehrer. 2008. "The Impact of Alternative Food for Education Programs on School Participation and Education Attainment in Northern Uganda." http://users.ox.ac.uk/~econ0274/downloads/Alderman_Gilligan_Lehrer_FFE__School_Participation.pdf.

Arnold, C., and T. Conway. 2011. "DFID Cash Transfers Evidence Paper." DFID Policy Division 2011, Department for International Development (DFID), London.

Bundy, D. 2005. "School Health and Nutrition: Policy and Programs." *Food and Nutrition Bulletin* 26 (2 suppl. 2): S186–92.

Bundy, D. 2011. "New Reasons Why School-Based Deworming Is Smart Development Policy." Posted on Education for Global Development, a World Bank blog about the power of investing in people.

Bundy, D., C. Burbano, M. Grosh, A. Gelli, M. Jukes, and L. Drake. 2009. *Rethinking School Feeding: Social Safety Nets, Child Development and the Education Sector.* Washington, DC: World Food Programme and the World Bank.

Coates, D. 2003. "Education Production Functions Using Instructional Time as an Input." *Education Economics* 11: 273–92.

Coutts, D. 1998. "How to Better Track Effective School Indicators. The Control Chart Techniques." *American Secondary Education* 27: 2–10.

Duclos, J. Y., P. Makdissi, and Q. Wodon. 2008. "Socially Efficient Tax Reforms." *International Economic Review* 49 (4): 1505–37.

Edstrom, J., H. Lucas, R. Sabates-Wheeler, and B. Simwaka. 2008. "A Study of the Outcomes of Take-Home Food Rations for Orphans and Vulnerable Children in Communities Affected by AIDS in Malawi: A Research Report." UNICEF ESARO, Nairobi.

FAO (Food and Agriculture Organisation of the United Nations). 2008. "The State of Food Insecurity in the World, 2008." FAO, Rome. http://www.fao.org/docrep/011/i0291e/i0291e00.htm.

Finn, J. D. 1989. "Withdrawing from School." *Review of Educational Research* 59: 117–42.

Foeken, D., S. O. Owuor, and A. M. Mwangi. 2007. "School Farming and School Feeding in Nakuru Town, Kenya: Practice and Potential." ASC Working Paper 76/2007, African Studies Centre, Leiden, the Netherlands.

Galasso, E., and M. Ravallion. 2005. "Decentralized Targeting of an Antipoverty Program." *Journal of Public Economics* 89: 705–27.

Galloway, R., E. Kristjansson, A. Gelli, U. Meir, F. Espejo, and D. Bundy. 2009. "School Feeding: Outcomes and Costs". Food and Nutrition Bulletin. June 30 (2): 171–182. Program for Appropriate Technology in Health, Washington, DC 2006, USA.

Galloway, R. 2010. "Developing Rations for Home Grown School Feeding." PCD Working Paper 214, Partnership for Child Development, London.

Gelb, A., and S. Majerowicz. 2011. "Oil for Uganda—or Ugandans? Can Cash Transfers Prevent the Resource Curse?" Working Paper 261, Center for Global Development, Washington, DC.

Gelli, A., U. Meir, and F. Espejo. 2007. "Does Provision of Food in School Increase Girls' Enrollment? Evidence from Schools in Sub-Saharan Africa." *Food and Nutrition Bulletin* 28 (2): 149–55.

Gottfried, M. A. 2009. "Evaluating the Relationship between Student Attendance and Achievement in Urban Elementary and Middle Schools: An Instrumental Variables Approach." *American Educational Research Journal* 20 (10): 1–32.

Hamdani, S. 2008. "Micronutrient Sprinkles to Address Multiple Deficiencies in School Age Children." World Food Programme School Feeding, Rome.

Jukes, M., J. Drake, and P. Bundy. 2008. *School Health, Nutrition and Education for All: Leveling the Playing Field*. Cambridge, MA: CABI Publishing.

Kain, J., R. Uauy, and M. Taibo. 2002. "Chile's School Feeding Programme: Targeting Experience." *Nutritional Research* 22: 599–608.

Kakwani, N., F. Soares, and H. H. Son. 2005. "Conditional Cash Transfers in African Countries." International Poverty Centre Working Paper, United Nations Development Programme, Brasilia.

Makdissi, P., and Q. Wodon. 2002. "Consumption Dominance Curves: Testing for the Impact of Indirect Tax Reforms on Poverty." *Economics Letters* 75: 227–35.

Miguel, E., and M. Kremer. 2004. "Worms: Identifying Impacts on Education and Health in the Presence of Treatment Externalities." *Econometrica* 72 (1): 159–217.

NFA (National Forestry Authority). 2009. "National Biomass Study." Technical Report, unpublished, NFA, Kampala, Uganda.

Pietzsch, S. 2011. "Unconditional Cash Transfers: Giving Choice to People in Need." Practice and Policy Notes, *Humanitarian Exchange* 49 (January): 19.

Pollitt, E., S. Cueto, and E. R. Jacoby. 1998. "Fasting and Cognition in Well and Undernourished Schoolchildren: A Review of Three Experimental Studies." *American Journal of Clinical Nutrition* 76 (4): 779S–84S.

Raimer, M. 2002. "Belize School Feeding Program" *Plenty Belize Summer Bulletin* 18 (2). http://www.plenty.org/pb18_2/feedingprog182.html.

Republic of Uganda. 2010. "National Development Plan (NDP), 2010/11–2014/15." National Planning Authority, Kampala.

Smithers, N. 2011. *The Importance of Stakeholder Ownership for Capacity Development Results*. Washington, DC: World Bank Institute.

Subbarao, K., A. Bonnerjee, J. Braithwaite, S. Carvalho, K. Ezemenari, C. Graham, and A. Thompson. 1997. *Safety Net Programs and Poverty Reduction: Lessons from Cross-Country Experience*. Directions in Development Series. Washington, DC: World Bank.

Tabor, S. 2002. "Assisting the Poor with Cash: Design and Implementation of Social Transfer Programs." Social Safety Net Primer Series. World Bank Institute, Washington, DC. http://info.worldbank.org/etools/docs/library/80703/Dc%202002/courses/dc2002/readings/taborcash.pdf.

UBOS (Uganda Bureau of Statistics). 2010. "Uganda National Household Survey, 2009/2010: Socio-Economic Module, Abridged Report." UBOS, Kampala.

———. 2011. *2011 Statistical Abstract*. Kampala: UBOS.

WFP (World Food Programme). 2006. *World Hunger Series 2006: Hunger and Learning*. Rome: WFP and Stanford University Press.

ECO-AUDIT
Environmental Benefits Statement

The World Bank is committed to preserving endangered forests and natural resources. The Office of the Publisher has chosen to print World Bank Studies and Working Papers on recycled paper with 30 percent postconsumer fiber in accordance with the recommended standards for paper usage set by the Green Press Initiative, a non-profit program supporting publishers in using fiber that is not sourced from endangered forests. For more information, visit www.greenpressinitiative.org.

In 2010, the printing of this book on recycled paper saved the following:

- 11 trees*
- 3 million Btu of total energy
- 1,045 lb. of net greenhouse gases
- 5,035 gal. of waste water
- 306 lb. of solid waste

_____

* 40 feet in height and 6–8 inches in diameter

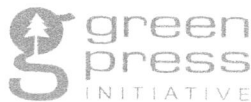

green press
INITIATIVE

www.ingramcontent.com/pod-product-compliance
Lightning Source LLC
Chambersburg PA
CBHW080332270325
41927CB00014B/3262